THE YOGA WAY:
FOOD FOR BODY, MIND & SPIRIT

by Sri Swami Satchidananda

*with a foreword by Dean Ornish, M.D. and
a special section on getting started
by Sandra McLanahan, M.D.*

Other Titles Available from Integral Yoga® Publications

Books by Sri Swami Satchidananda

The Yoga Sutras of Patanjali

Beyond Words

The Living Gita

Yoga Affirmations Coloring Book

To Know Your Self

Integral Yoga Hatha

The Golden Present

The Breath of Life

Books About Sri Swami Satchidananda

Boundless Giving:
    The Life and Service of Sri Swami Satchidananda

Sri Swami Satchidananda: Portrait of a Modern Sage

Sri Swami Satchidananda: Apostle of Peace

Sri Swami Satchidananda:
    A Yoga Master's Early Days in India and Sri Lanka

Other Titles

A Vision of Peace:
    The Interfaith Teachings of Sri Swami Satchidananda

Awakening: Aspiration to Realization through Integral Yoga

Bound to Be Free: The Liberating Power of Prison Yoga

Dictionary of Sanskrit Names

Enlightening Tales As Told By Sri Swami Satchidananda

Everybody's Vegan Cookbook

Hatha Yoga for Kids by Kids

Inside the Yoga Sutras

LOTUS: Light Of Truth Universal Shrine

Lotus Prayer Book

Sparkling Together

Yogaville Recipes

THE YOGA WAY:
FOOD FOR BODY, MIND & SPIRIT

by Sri Swami Satchidananda

with a foreword by Dean Ornish, M.D. and
a special section on getting started
by Sandra McLanahan, M.D.

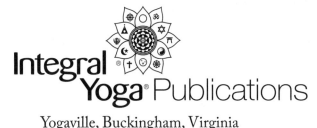

Yogaville, Buckingham, Virginia
www.integralyoga.org

Library of Congress Cataloging-in-Publication Data

Satchidananda, Swami

  The Yoga Way.

  Bibliography: p.

  1. Vegetarianism. I. Title.

TX392.S28   1986   613.2'62   86-2974

ISBN 978-0-932040-01-5

Integral Yoga® Publications
108 Yogaville Way, Virginia 23921, U.S.A.

Printed in the United States of America.

FOREWORD

I welcome this opportunity to write the foreword to this important book, as awareness is the first step in healing.

For almost four decades, my colleagues and I at the non-profit Preventive Medicine Research Institute and the University of California, San Francisco have conducted clinical research proving the many benefits of comprehensive lifestyle changes.

This is the era of lifestyle medicine—that is, changes in diet and lifestyle to treat and even *reverse* the progression of many of the most common chronic diseases as well as to help prevent them. These include:

- a whole foods, plant-based diet (naturally low in fat and refined carbohydrates) like the one described in this book;

- stress management techniques (including Yoga and meditation); moderate exercise (such as walking);

- and social support and community (love and intimacy).

In short—eat well, move more, stress less, and love more.

This lifestyle program is based on what I learned from Sri Swami Satchidananda, a renowned spiritual teacher with whom I had the privilege of studying for 30 years beginning in 1972. He made a profound difference in my life and in the lives of millions of others.

He taught me the importance of addressing the underlying *causes* of many chronic diseases. As he often said, "For most people, our natural state is to be easeful and peaceful. We are born with ease until we disturb it by making unhealthy lifestyle choices and become dis-eased. We are born fine until we allow ourselves to become de-fined."

In other words, these diet and lifestyle changes don't *bring* us health and well-being. Rather, they help us to identify and change diet, behaviors, and perceptions that disturb our inner peace, joy, and well-being, thereby allowing our bodies' exquisite healing mechanisms to work and heal optimally.

Many people tend to think of advances in medicine as high-tech and expensive, such as a new drug, laser, or surgical procedure. We often have a hard time believing that something as simple as comprehensive lifestyle changes can make such a powerful difference in our lives—but they often do.

In our research, we've used high-tech, expensive, state-of-the-art scientific measure to prove the power of these simple, low-tech, and low-cost interventions. These randomized controlled trials and other studies have been published in the leading peer-reviewed medical and scientific journals.

In addition to *preventing* many chronic diseases, these comprehensive lifestyle changes can often *reverse* the progression of these illnesses.

We proved, for the first time, that lifestyle changes alone can reverse the progression of even severe coronary heart disease. There was even more reversal after five years than after one year and 2.5 times fewer cardiac events. We also found that these lifestyle changes can reverse type 2 diabetes and may slow, stop, or even reverse the progression of early-stage prostate cancer.

Changing lifestyle actually changes your genes—turning on genes that keep you healthy, and turning off genes that promote heart disease, prostate cancer, breast cancer, and diabetes—over 500 genes in only three months. People often say, "Oh, it's all in my genes, there's not much I can do about it." But there is. Knowing that changing lifestyle changes our genes is often very motivating—not to blame, but to empower. Our genes are a predisposition, but our genes are not our fate.

Our latest research found that these diet and lifestyle changes may even lengthen telomeres, the ends of our chromosomes that control aging. As our telomeres get longer, our life gets longer. This was the first controlled study showing that any intervention may begin to reverse aging on a cellular level by lengthening telomeres. And the more people adhered to these lifestyle recommendations, the longer their telomeres became.

This is a different approach to personalized medicine. It's not like there was one set of dietary recommendations for reversing heart disease, a different one for reversing diabetes, and yet another for changing your genes or lengthening your telomeres. In all of our studies, people were asked to consume a whole foods plant-based diet like the one described in this book. Because it's pleasurable, it's sustainable.

And it's not all or nothing. What matters most is your *overall* way of eating and living. In all of our studies, we found that the more people changed their diet and lifestyle, the more they improved and the better they felt—at any age. If you indulge yourself one day, eat healthier the next. If you don't have time to meditate for an hour, do it for a minute. The more you do, the more you improve. And quickly.

And what's good for you is good for our planet. To the degree we transition toward a whole foods plant-based diet, it not only makes a difference in our own lives, it also makes a difference in the lives of many others across the globe as well.

The crises in global warming, health care costs, and energy resources can feel overwhelming: "What can I do as one person to make a difference?" This may lead to inaction, depression, and even nihilism.

However, when we realize that something as primal as what we choose to put in our mouths each day makes a difference in all three of these crises, it empowers us and imbues these choices with meaning. If it's meaningful, then it's sustainable—and *a meaningful life is a longer life.*

Health Crisis

More than 86% of the $3.2 trillion in annual U.S. health care costs (mostly sick-care costs) are from chronic diseases which can often be prevented and even reversed by eating a plant-based diet, at a fraction of the costs.

For example, in the European Prospective Investigation into Cancer and Nutrition (EPIC) study, patients who adhered to healthy dietary principles (low meat consumption and high intake of fruits, vegetables, and whole-grain bread), never smoked, were not overweight, and had at least 30 minutes a day of physical activity had a 78% lower overall risk of developing a chronic disease. This included a 93% reduced risk of diabetes, an 81% lower risk of heart attacks, a 50% reduction in risk of stroke, and a 36% overall reduction in risk of cancer, compared with participants without these healthy factors.

It's not just low-fat vs. low-carb. A study found that *animal protein dramatically increases the risk of premature death independent of fat and carbs.* In a study of over 6,000 people, those aged 50-65 who reported eating diets high in animal protein had a 75% increase in overall mortality, a 400% increase in cancer deaths, and a 500% increase in type 2 diabetes during the following 18 years.

Only 5% of people account for 80% of health care costs. Our research has shown that when comprehensive lifestyle changes are offered as *treatment* (not just as prevention), sometimes in combination with drugs or surgery, significant cost savings occur in the first year because the biological mechanisms that control our health and well-being are so dynamic.

For example, Highmark Blue Cross Blue Shield found that overall health care costs were reduced by 50% in the first year when people with heart disease or risk factors went through our lifestyle program in 24 hospitals and clinics in West Virginia, Pennsylvania, and Nebraska. In patients who spent more than

$25,000 on health care in the prior year, costs were reduced 400% in the following year. In another study, Mutual of Omaha found that they saved $30,000 per patient in the first year in those who went through our lifestyle program.

Because of these findings, we are grateful that Medicare began covering our program of lifestyle medicine in 2010. If it's reimbursable, it's sustainable. (For more information, please go to www.ornish.com.)

Global Warming Crisis

Many people are surprised to learn that animal agribusiness generates more greenhouse gases than all forms of transportation combined. The livestock sector generates more greenhouse gas emissions than the entire global transportation chain as measured in carbon dioxide equivalent (18% vs. 13.5%). More recent estimates are that these numbers are even higher—that livestock and their byproducts may actually account for more than 50% of annual worldwide greenhouse gas emissions (at least 32.6 billion tons of carbon dioxide per year).

It is also responsible for 37% of all the human-induced methane, which is 23 times more toxic to the ozone layer than carbon dioxide, as well as generating 65% of the human related nitrous oxide, which has 296 times the global warming potential of carbon dioxide. Nitrous oxide and methane mostly come from manure, and 56 billion "food animals" produce a lot of manure each day.

Also, livestock now use 30% of the earth's entire land surface, mostly for permanent pasture but also including 33% of global arable land to produce feed for them. As forests are cleared to create new pastures for livestock, it is a major driver of deforestation: some 70% of forests in the Amazon have been turned over to grazing.

Energy Crisis

It takes more than 10 times the amount of resources to produce a pound of meat-based protein as plant-based protein. Thus, if more people shifted from eating a meat-based to a plant-based diet, that would provide significantly more resources to feed the hungry and heal our planet.

More than half of U.S. grain and nearly 40% of world grain is being fed to livestock rather than being consumed directly by humans. In the United States, more than 8 billion livestock are maintained, which eat about seven times as much grain as is consumed directly by the entire U.S. population.

Producing 2.2 lbs. of fresh beef requires about 28.6 lbs. of grain and 66 lbs. of forage. This much grain and forage requires more than 11,360 gallons of water. As Swami Satchidananda often said, we have enough food to feed everyone if enough people would consume a whole foods plant-based diet.

We're always making choices in our lives. If what we gain is more than what we give up, then it's sustainable. Because these underlying biological mechanisms are so dynamic, if you eat and live this way for a few weeks, you're likely to feel so much better, so quickly, you'll find that these are choices worth making—not from fear of dying but joy of living.

The Harvard Health Professionals Study and the Harvard Nurses Health Study followed more than 37,000 men and 83,000 women for almost 3 million person-years. They found that consumption of both processed and unprocessed red meat is associated with an increased risk of premature mortality from all causes as well as from cardiovascular disease, cancer, and type 2 diabetes.

And it's not just the arteries in your heart that get clogged on a diet high in red meat. Erectile dysfunction—impotence— is *significantly higher* in meat eaters. In men 40 to 70, over *half* report problems with erectile dysfunction.

Good news: in the *Massachusetts Male Aging Study*, eating a diet rich in fruit, vegetables, whole grains, and fish—with fewer red and processed meat and refined grains— significantly decreased the likelihood of impotence. It's not just your heart that gets more blood flow when you eat a whole foods plant-based diet.

Changing your diet is not all or nothing. Start with a meatless Monday (or Tuesday or Wednesday). To the degree you move in this direction, there is a corresponding benefit. You'll look better and feel better, have hotter love and a cooler planet.

Now *that's* sustainable.

To the degree we choose to eat a plant-based diet, we free up tremendous amounts of resources that can benefit many others as well as ourselves. We have enough food in the world to feed everyone if enough people were to eat lower on the food chain. I find this very inspiring and motivating. When we can act more compassionately, it helps our hearts as well.

And the only side-effects are good ones.

Dean Ornish, M.D.
Founder and President, Preventive Medicine Research Institute
Clinical Professor of Medicine, University of California, San Francisco.
Author, *The Spectrum* and *Dr. Dean Ornish's Program for Reversing Heart Disease*
www.ornish.com

PREFACE

The author of this book, Sri Swami Satchidananda, is well known as a modern day Yoga Master and founder of Integral Yoga. As a native of India, Yoga's original home, Sri Swamiji grew up steeped in yogic tradition. Having achieved the experience of "the peace that passeth all understanding," he traveled the world over, invited by groups and institutions, sharing the teachings of Yoga, including some of its ramifications in the fields of health, world peace, and religious unity.

People often asked him, "Do you have a prescription for a healthy diet?" His gentle and non-dogmatic answer was, "I would never want to give a 'prescription' for a healthy diet, because one person's nectar is another's poison. Constitutions vary, lifestyles vary, so each one has to decide what is best for him or her. But I would generally recommend any diet that would not deposit toxins into the system, that would be easily digested, and would give enough nutrition."

But, seeing how active and healthy Swami Satchidananda was—and knowing him to be a lifelong vegetarian—the questioning often turned to his personal choice, that of vegetarianism. He had this to say about his own experience:

"I have been a vegetarian all of my life. I work day and night. I travel twenty days out of the month. One day I am in Virginia, the next I might be in Dallas, Texas, the day after that in London. Almost every day I am lecturing and meeting people, and with all that I eat only once a day and only vegetarian food. And when I am not traveling, I do manual work also. I drive a tractor, operate heavy equipment, ride a horse. My perspiration is always clean, sometimes sweet-smelling, like sandalwood. In fact, I have tried going for an entire month without taking a bath and I never smelled bad. I don't fall sick; I never even get the 'common cold' or headache. At one time a doctor wanted to test the health of my internal organs. He found that my kidneys and heart were those of a twenty-five year old. My chiropractor says I have the spine of an eighteen year old. I sleep very little, only a few hours a night."

This testimonial may inspire us, and yet leave us with many questions about vegetarianism and diet. In the first two parts of this book Sri Swamiji shares his thoughts on many aspects of vegetarianism, from issues of physical health and questions of morality to a discussion of the effects of meat diet and vegetarian diet upon our minds. He also tackles psychological and moral issues such as dealing with non-vegetarian family members and even dealing with insect pests on home-grown vegetables. And finally, there is a compendium of his advice on specific issues pertaining to Yogic diet.

~Reverend Vidya Vonne
Editor: Parts I–II

PLEASE NOTE: The suggestions made in this book are based on the authors' own experiences and are not meant to be a substitute for professional medical advice.

ACKNOWLEDGMENTS

Integral Yoga® Publications would like to thank Rev. Vidya Vonne for her fine efforts in compiling, organizing, and editing the material in Parts I through II of this book. Her untimely passing in 2017 only makes her contributions over the years more treasured.

Thank you to Sandra Amrita McLanahan, M.D. for contributing the section on helping beginning vegetarians and vegans get started.

Despite an incredibly busy schedule, Dean Ornish, M.D. wrote the Foreword for this book and we deeply appreciate this and all his pioneering work in the field of Lifestyle Medicine.

Our great thanks to Carole Kalyani Baral, M.S. for her service in helping to vision this project, in compiling the information contained in the Making the Transition and Resources sections and in contributing to the Yogic Diet section.

Our special thanks to Swami Karunananda for her guidance in the preparation of the section on Yogic Diet and to Rev. Sandra Kumari de Sachy, Ed.D. for also contributing to this section.

Our great appreciation to Satchidananda Ashram–Yogaville and the Integral Yoga Institute of San Francisco for sharing some delicious and healthful recipes in the recipe section of this book.

Our sincere appreciation to Colleen Vimala Patterson for the cover design, Alain Shiva Hervé for the book layout, and Rev. Prem Anjali, who served as a contributor to several of the sections and also as project manager.

We are deeply grateful to Mr. & Mrs. Harry Wadhwani, Mr. & Mrs. Chandru Wadhwani, and Reverend Sivani Alderman for all their generous support of the wisdom teachings of Sri Swami Satchidananda. This support, over many years, makes it possible to share these teachings far and wide. We know that Sri Swamiji's blessings are with them always.

CONTENTS

DESSERT RECIPES

QUICK FIX, KID FRIENDLY MINI-MEAL AND SNACK RECIPES

ABOUT THE AUTHOR

ABOUT THE CONTRIBUTORS

PART I:

WHY SHOULD I BE A VEGETARIAN?

by Sri Swami Satchidananda

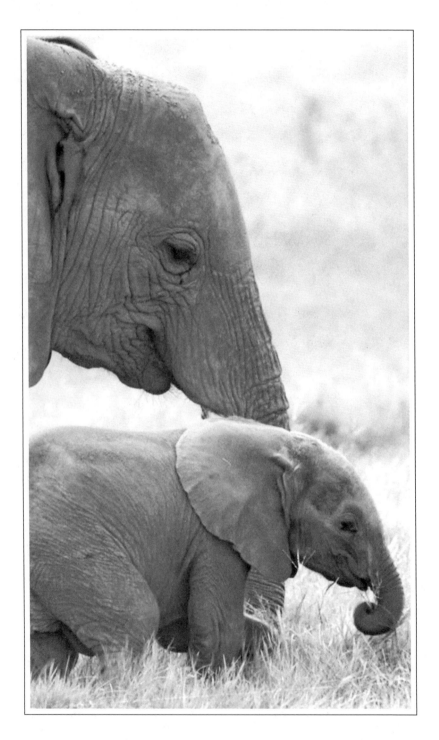

CHAPTER 1:

INTRODUCTION TO VEGETARIAN LIFE

"Why should someone want to become a vegetarian?" Many, many people have asked me this question. And in this scientific age most people want to see some proof of the benefit of something before they try it. So I would like to share with you some of the history regarding one study with which I was involved.

In 1977, I was invited to speak at the Baylor College of Medicine in Houston, Texas. More coronary bypass operations were performed in the medical center there than anywhere else in the United States. The students and doctors were very interested in my talk about vegetarian diet and Yoga.

One of the medical doctors at Baylor at that time, was a student of mine named Dean Ornish. He wanted to study the effect of vegetarian diet and Yoga on coronary heart disease. He had been working with a group of patients who had acute problems, many of which could not be corrected by surgery.

The Plaza Hotel in Houston generously donated one month's use of ten rooms for the study. Some of the patients spent the entire time there; others went to work during the day and came "home" to the hotel at night. All of them were put on a program of a strict vegetarian diet, simple Yoga postures and breathing exercises, progressive deep relaxation, and healing visualization.

After one month, most of the patients demonstrated substantial improvement. Many became pain free. Many of those who wanted to go back to work full-time were able to do so. Most important, tests indicated that the heart was able to receive an increased blood flow through such treatment. This had never been documented in such a way before.

Later, we repeated the study in a more definitive way. In this second study, forty-eight heart patient volunteers were randomly divided into two equal groups. One group had the program of a vegetarian diet and Yoga for three and a half weeks; the other group received only their usual medical care during the same period.

When tested after the program, the vegetarian group showed substantial improvements. These patients experienced a 91 percent reduction of angina (chest pain), increased exercise capability, reduced blood pressure, and reduced cholesterol levels. Nuclear cardiology tests indicated that each one's heart was beating and pumping blood more effectively. In contrast, the control group showed none of these improvements.

Other scientific studies have also been conducted on vegetarianism and have also showed very positive effects. Why is this? There are many reasons, some of which I will present on the following pages. We should know, however, that health considerations are not the only arguments in favor of a vegetarian diet. We can look, too, from the points of view of philosophy, religion, ethics, ecology, and economics.

We can consider what kind of foods our bodies are physiologically designed for. And for those interested in the effects of food on our minds, we can look at what kind of diet is most conducive to our mental well-being. Considering even one of these points is likely to make us think more seriously about adopting a vegetarian diet. When we look at all of them, the evidence becomes quite convincing.

So, for the sake of our physical and mental well-being, and for the well-being of our beloved planet Earth, I present the following facts about vegetarianism. It is my sincere hope and prayer that this information might help open your mind to new possibilities for a healthier, happier life.

CHAPTER 2:

OUR NATURAL DIET

Let us first consider the question, "What is the natural diet for human beings?" When we look at the diet of mammals, we find two major groups: the flesh-eating animals, such as dogs, cats, tigers and lions; and the vegetarian animals, such as cows, bulls, horses, camels, monkeys—and even the largest land animal, the elephant.

Comparing their physical features, the flesh-eating animals have long teeth to tear the raw animal flesh from the bones, while the vegetarian animals all have flat teeth for grinding vegetable food. Meat-eating animals have rough tongues to lick the flesh from the bone and sharp, strong claws to catch and kill their prey, while vegetarian animals do not. The meat-eaters also have excellent night vision for hunting, while the vegetarians have more difficulty seeing after dusk.

These are just the external features that can be seen. There are others, which we cannot see. The intestines of meat-eating animals are only about two to three times their body length. That means that the meat they eat can pass through their systems quickly before it putrefies.

Vegetarian animals' intestines are about six or seven times their bodies' length, because their systems need not push the food through so rapidly. The vegetarians have a different pH in their saliva and their stomachs than the meat-eaters; vegetarians also have digestive enzymes in their saliva, and begin digesting while the food is still in the mouth, while meat-eaters gulp their food without much chewing.

Now let us look at the human animal. Human beings have flat, grinding teeth—like the vegetarians. They do not have the rough tongues or sharp claws of the meat-eaters. Humans also have more difficulty seeing after dusk. Their intestines are about twenty-six feet long or six to seven times their body's length—like the vegetarians. The pH of their saliva is similar to vegetarians', and it contains digestive enzymes. So the evidence seems indisputable: by physical design, we are certainly vegetarian animals.

You might argue, "What about the Eskimos whose diet is primarily meat? How can you tell them that they are vegetarians by nature and should give up meat? They would starve!" I would never advocate vegetarian diet in such an environment where even grass does not grow. If vegetable food will not grow, certainly we must eat animals. Why stop there? If nothing else is available, people will even eat each other. We have seen this happen at various times in the world.

It may be difficult for us to admit, but it is a fact. We have to survive. But when we *can* get the food most suited to our natures, certainly we should do so. If you still want to use the Eskimos as an example, you should note that the average life span of an Inuit Eskimo is twelve to fifteen years less than the average Canadian and lower than the other three indigenous groups of Canada. Compare this with the life span of the Hunzas of Pakistan, whose diet is primarily vegetarian. Recorded ages of 110 are not uncommon among their population.

Food: Its Effects on Body and Mind

If you want to see the differences between flesh-eating and vegetarian animals very clearly, go to the zoo. Look carefully at the different animals. The meat-eating animals all need to be caged: the tigers, the lions, the leopards. Even inside their cages, they are restless, pacing endlessly back and forth. They are fierce and aggressive. And you may even hesitate to go near their cages because they smell so bad. Everything that comes out of their bodies smells foul.

The vegetarian animals, on the other hand, are calm and gentle; they are not frightening. Often they do not even need to be caged; they walk slowly, peacefully. They can be allowed to roam around freely. And their bodies do not smell bad. You can even put your nose right into the mouth of a cow and not find any foul smell. It is the same with their perspiration, their urine, their excrement. If you have been to India, you might know that cow dung is used to clean the floors there. Pick up a piece of cow dung and smell it; there is no bad smell at all. Can you comfortably smell the dung of a dog?

Why should flesh-eating animals smell bad while vegetarian ones do not? It is because of the food they eat. That's why almost all meat-eating people cannot expose their armpits without embarrassment! They have to constantly spray deodorants to cover up the foul smell, because what they eat comes out through their pores. If you are a strict vegetarian with a clean diet, your perspiration will not smell bad. Many meat-eating people will never take off their shoes in the presence of others because their feet smell so bad. If you are a vegetarian you need not worry about such things. Even if you do not take a bath for ten days, your body will not smell bad.

So, in both physical and mental conditions, carnivores differ from herbivores. As you know, mostly all soldiers in wartime eat a diet high in meat. If you give them yogic food they will not fight. We feed them meat, expecting them to act like wild animals. However, some of the commanders who direct them are vegetarians because they have to think clearly.

When I am asked, "Is there any way of stopping war?," I often answer, "Send the soldiers barrels of fruits and nuts; stop the war 'drum and rum,' play some symphonic music." The meat, the war drum, and the liquor all affect the minds of the soldiers. It makes them *rajasic*—restless, warlike. Without all that they would just throw away their guns and sit and meditate. That is the power of food and of sound vibration.

CHAPTER 3:
HEALTH CONSIDERATIONS

Live vs. Dead Food

We have looked at the effects of vegetarian diet on the mind and at some of its physical effects. But there is much more that can be said about the relationship between vegetarian diet and health. The vegetarian diet is the best diet known for promoting good health.

A diet of fruit, vegetables, grains, legumes, nuts and seeds will not leave a lot of toxins in our systems. It is the animal matter that leaves so much toxic material. Why? Because the minute you kill an animal, its body, its corpse, starts to decay. Once the animal is killed, it is dead matter. We are literally eating dead matter.

This is not the case with vegetables. They may dehydrate, but it will be a very long time before they decay. Eat half of a vegetable and plant the other half. It will grow again. It is still a living organism. Take the stem of a spinach plant, cut it into ten parts. Eat the leaves, but plant the pieces of stem and you will get ten new spinach plants. Can you do that with a lamb? Can you eat its leg and then make the other parts grow into another lamb? No, because it is dead matter.

Toxicity of Meat

People sometimes think it's possible to find healthy animals to eat. But even if the veterinarian has certified that an animal is healthy before slaughter, at the time of killing what happens to its system? What happens to *your* system when you are frightened? Adrenalin courses throughout the body, affecting every cell. The same thing happens within an animal. At the moment of slaughter, all kinds of undesirable toxins and hormones get splashed into the body. Where do they go after that? Nowhere; they remain in the meat that comes to your table.

Because our intestines are so long, approximately twenty-two to twenty-six feet, the decayed flesh cannot be digested and pass through before it putrefies. Although the body tries to filter out the toxins through the eliminative system (the perspiration, the breath, etc.), all of the toxins are not eliminated. It's these wastes remaining in the system that thicken the arteries with cholesterol, often causing atherosclerosis, and eventually high blood pressure, strokes and heart attacks.

It's the elimination of these toxins that causes foul perspiration odor. If everyone were to become a vegetarian, we could close all the deodorant factories. We often see television commercials in which a young man comes up to talk to a young woman, only to have her make a face and run away. So he goes and sprays something in his mouth and then all the ladies come flocking around him! How long can people live on a spray? If they really want to attract others, let them live on pure vegetarian food. The perspiration of a person who lives on pure food will have a scent like flowers; it might even be sweet, like jasmine or sandalwood.

When such a person moves his or her bowels, there will be no need to wash or use toilet paper. Don't we see this even in a goat? The excrement comes out very smoothly in small black balls covered with a kind of white coating; it does not even soil the goat's body. We can have that kind of elimination. When you eat the proper food in the proper quantity, your excreta is formulated well; it passes through in softish balls and never smells bad. If it smells or is clay-like or too loose, something is wrong in the stomach or intestines.

Protein

Many people are concerned about getting enough protein. It's true that there is a lot of protein in meat, but we don't need that concentrated a protein in our systems. It isn't a simple form of protein, but one that is very concentrated, very rich. Even the meat-eating animals try to eat only vegetarian animals. Meat-eating humans also eat only vegetarian animals. They would never eat a carnivorous animal.

Our protein should be as close to its natural source as possible. A vegetarian animal gives us better protein than a meat-eating one; eating the vegetables themselves is better still. There is plenty of protein in beans and lentils, in avocados, nuts and seeds. There it is found in a simple form that is easy to digest and assimilate.

Flexibility, Ease, & Physical Strength

Vegetarians have bodies that are healthier and more supple than the bodies of meat-eaters. They also have much less tension in their bodies. The moment a person changes from a meat diet, he or she will feel a lightness and a release of tension. I have heard this over and over again. Yoga postures and other forms of exercise become easier, and sometimes long-standing complaints—such as insomnia or nervousness—disappear.

Some people are concerned about how they will be able to keep up their strength without having meat in their diet. I would recommend that they ask an elephant. The elephants are the biggest and strongest animals in the world, and they are pure vegetarians. Some clever minds will argue, "But a tiger can kill an elephant." That is true. Both tigers and elephants are strong. But what kind of strength does the tiger have? Killing strength. What kind of strength does the elephant have? Pulling strength. It can pull ten huge logs at a time. Can you tie a log to the tail of a tiger and get it to pull it? No. So what kind of strength is more useful to us: restless, killing strength or steady, pulling strength?

CHAPTER 4:

YOGIC VALUES

Ahimsa: Non-Violence

Many people are concerned about the violence in our society and about the threat that violence poses to the very existence of our planet. Our meat diet is a part of that violence. We should think about such things, and about adopting a policy of *ahimsa*.

Ahimsa is a Sanskrit word that means non-violence. Following *ahimsa* doesn't simply mean not killing. We cannot live without destroying other lives. When you eat vegetables, you are killing, destroying something. Even if you don't eat anything, you kill.

Do you know how many bacteria you kill each time you take a drink of water? Millions. If it is a matter of avoiding *killing* alone, I would advocate eating meat. Why? Simple mathematical calculations: If you want to eat spinach, how many plants must you kill? Certainly ten or twenty for even one meal. But how many people can eat from just one sheep? Say ten people. If every life you take is one "sin," which is better? Certainly, killing one sheep would be better. So it's not killing we are talking about here. We are talking about non-violence.

What do we mean by violence? If I do something to you and you feel hurt, my act was violent. Causing pain is violence. If we want to be non-violent, our food should come with as little pain as possible. Many people would say, "But plants are alive, too. They feel pain if we pluck and eat them. So why give up meat if not causing pain is the idea?"

Yes, plants have life; animals have life; human beings have life; even an atom has life. In having life we are all equal. But in the expression of consciousness the plant is not as developed as the animal, nor the animal as developed as the human being. Human beings are bestowed with discrimination; it's human beings who even think of all this, who think of comparing themselves with other beings. Animals don't compare themselves with humans. Plants are even less developed in the expression of their consciousness. The more developed the expression of consciousness in a particular form of life, the more pain is felt when you destroy it. Cutting off the branch of a tree causes less pain than cutting off the limb of an animal. Many studies show that plants *do* experience pain; but still, we believe it's not as much as the animals experience.

Here is an analogy that might help illustrate this principle. Imagine a classroom of thirty students with a teacher standing in the front of the room, writing on the blackboard. Somewhere in one of the rows two of the students are talking loudly. One is the brightest student in the class. Normally he would not be doing such a thing, but today somehow the other fellow drew him into it. The other boy is "number one" at the other end. He is the worst student and has no interest in studying at all. He simply came to the classroom because it was even worse at home. So they are both talking. The teacher looks at them and yells, "Hey, you fools, what are you doing there?"

Which of the two do you think would feel most hurt by being called a fool in front of the whole class? The "number one" brilliant boy. The other one might just shrug it off, thinking "I've heard it many times . . ." Or he might even feel proud: "Finally, the teacher noticed me, paid some attention to me!" But the first one would say, "I'm sorry, I won't do it again!" He might even burst into tears because he's never been addressed like that before. How can the same word create two different feelings in two individuals? One had a sharper, more evolved mind. The other one had a duller mind. It all depends on the development of the consciousness. The bright boy's consciousness was more developed. The other's was still a little dull. So the same action will hurt the evolved soul more than the unevolved soul.

Now, let us apply this analogy to the animals and the vegetables. The animals are supposed to have evolved a little bit more in their consciousness than the plants. The Hindu scriptures say, "Consciousness sleeps in mineral life, dreams in plant life, awakens in animal life." In animals we see instinct functioning. Then, in the human level, we see intelligence, and finally in the superhuman—the yogi—intuition functions. It's all the same consciousness functioning at different levels.

It's with this awareness that we say the animals feel pain more than the plants. Since we still have to eat to live, but we want to reduce the pain-giving, the violence, where should we go? To the plants. And if you want to be still less violent, you can think even further. There have been many saints in India who said, "No, I cannot even pluck an unripe fruit." They live on fruits that have already fallen from the tree. If you try to pluck an unripe apple, the tree will resist you: "No, no, don't take it; I'm not ready yet." It is still "cooking" the apple. If by force you pluck it anyway, it bleeds, it weeps. You are hurting the tree. Wait until the fruit comes off in your hand by the mere touch. Then you are truly non-violent.

Moreover, after you eat the fruit, you throw the seed somewhere. That is nature's way of spreading. The fruit is your bait. "Come on, eat my flesh, but throw my seeds somewhere else. Let me spread out." You are not hurting the plant. On the other hand, you are expanding its species. You cannot do that with animals. You cannot eat the thigh of a cow and throw the head somewhere and make another cow grow.

Compassion & Moral Accountability

Where is our *karuna*, our compassion? What is happening to our hearts? If you have even once seen pictures of the young seals being killed for their fur, you will never wear fur again. In the same way, if you once saw how the animals die in the slaughterhouse, you would never want to eat meat again. Just because the killing is done by somebody else, somewhere else, does not mean that the karma, the responsibility, is not yours. You are contributing to their actions, and you share their karma.

Suppose tomorrow all the butchers were to say, "We are not going to kill for your sake anymore. If you want to eat an animal, you kill it." How many of you are ready to bring a lamb into your kitchen—the mother holding one leg, the father holding another, the son cutting it open while it screams and yells in pain, its blood splashing everywhere, all the fecal matter coming out—and then clean up all the blood and filth, cut it up, and eat it? No. When it's all wrapped up in nice cellophane, with no blood, no smell, just sitting in the supermarket case, then it seems all right to you.

When people do kill the animals themselves, seeing their blood and hearing their cries, eventually their hearts forget to be compassionate. They no longer see the pain they are causing. Some so-called compassionate people think, "If you chop their heads quickly before they even realize that they are going to die, it is humane." That is not so. Even miles away, hours before the slaughter, they know. You don't have to see them, nor do they have to see you. It is direct thought transference. They know that someone is coming to kill them.

We hear of so many organizations dedicated to saving pets. Members will go to court to save the life of a cat. Yet, those same people will kill hundreds of calves and cows for their parties. What is the difference between the cat's life and the cow's life? Every day so many animals are killed for food. What is the difference? "Cruelty toward animals . . ." these people cry; but why have they not extended that to our lambs, to our cows?

We are destroying the hearts and souls of millions of animals. We think we can get away without facing the karma for this, but we cannot. The Bible says, "Thou shalt not kill." We interpret that as thou shalt not *murder*—meaning only our fellow human beings. You can kill animals but you cannot kill a person because that is "murder." If you kill a person, you are taken to court; if you kill an animal, nobody will take you to court for that. But there is always God's court. God puts us into a bodily "prison" by creating problems within our own systems.

Why do you think that there are more people labeled insane here in the United States than anywhere else in the world? Every half hour someone goes insane. Every twenty minutes somebody commits suicide. We have the greatest number of cancer patients, the greatest number of heart patients. Why? It is our karma and we are paying. Whatever we do to other living beings comes back to us. That is the Nature's law. Nobody can save us from that. What you sow you have to reap. Instead of eating animals, we should learn to love them, but not to kill and eat them. When you die you have a graveyard somewhere. But, when they die, where is their graveyard? In your stomach.

We say we want a loving world, a peaceful world; but we cannot cultivate that love if negative vibrations get into us. One way in which we can bring negative vibrations into ourselves is through our food. That is why food should come to us as an offering of love.

Whatever we eat should be the product of love. When I say a loving offering, I don't mean that someone cooks a nice chicken soup or broiled steak and then offers it to you lovingly. The question is, "Did the animal who died to make that steak love you?" I don't think that any animal would die lovingly for you. Will a cow come and say, "Oh, you seem to be very weak and hungry, would you like my thigh for a soup? Take it." No, you have to kill it, destroy it.

In the same way, when you catch a fish, it does not come willingly. You have to cheat the fish by throwing a worm. Every time you catch a fish you are literally deceiving it. It's as if you are saying, "Come on, my friend, I will feed you." But when it comes to you, you hook it and kill it. Could you say that it is a love offering? The animals we kill hate us. If our food brings hatred, we cannot develop love.

You do not know how many thousands of animals will worship you if you become a vegetarian. You can be certain of that. A great South Indian saint Thiruvalluvar said, "If a person refrains from killing to eat, such a one will be worshipped by all the creatures of the world." It is true. Even a wild dog will wag its tail at you. The animals will feel that you are a non-violent person. Do not think that only the human beings have telecommunication. The animals have their own media, and fortunately *their* media carries the good news as well as the bad. If you have saved the life of another animal somewhere—it need not be even of the same species—the other animals will know, "You saved my brother or sister over there."

So eating the products of violence brings a violent vibration to the mind. You are what you eat; don't forget that. Your food should be a gift of love because the vibrations with which food comes to us will affect us. I will tell you a story about this—a true story.

Once, in India, a swami was invited to a rich man's house for a nice lunch. Normally, when the swami goes, a few disciples go with him. So they all went there and had a sumptuous lunch. It was served on beautiful silver plates, with silver cutlery, because the host was a very rich man. At the end of the meal, the swami blessed the man and his family, said goodbye, and left the house with his disciples.

They had been walking for about half a mile when one disciple, the youngest one, came running to the swami, "Swamiji, Swamiji, I made a terrible mistake!" The swami asked him, "What mistake is that?"

"Oh, I'm even ashamed to tell you, because I have never done anything like this before!"

"It's all right," the swami answered. "Don't worry; tell me." The disciple's hand was shaking as he pulled a silver spoon from his pocket. He said, "I took this from the man's house!" The swami smiled at him and said, "All right, you are still young; you are a beginner in spiritual practice. You will become strong as time goes on. Now, take it back and apologize; we will wait for you."

The other disciples questioned the swami: "Why were you so lenient with him? Don't you think you should be more strict?" The swami said, "No, it's not entirely his mistake."

"He stole the spoon, and you say it's not his mistake?!" Finally the swami explained, "Do you know the fellow who fed us, the rich man? He collected all that money through theft. He was formerly a banker, and he used to overcharge his customers. So, in a way, he is a thief. When he fed us with his food the vibrations of a thief also came with the food. You are all a little older and stronger, so it did not affect you. But he was affected by that vibration, and so he took the spoon."

It is a true story. I know the people involved very well. What does it mean? The fellow was a thief and had bought the food that he served that day with money that had been gained fraudulently. The food had that vibration. If you understand this, how careful you will be about how you get your food. Not all food is clean. It should come to you in a clean way and with a good heart. So think of this in the light of the animal food that you eat.

"But Jesus Ate Meat . . ."

Sometimes my Christian friends bring up the argument, "But Jesus ate meat and fish." My answer is: Jesus walked on water; Jesus accepted crucifixion. Are you ready to do that? "Oh, I'm not like Jesus in *that* way," they say. We just choose what we want to follow. We point out great saints and sages: "He did it, she did it, why shouldn't I?"

Here is an example of why. Once the great Hindu saint Acharya Shankara was walking with his students. It was a hot day and he felt thirsty. So he stopped a person who was coming from the other direction with a pot of some liquid.

"I'm thirsty, will you give me something to drink?" The man hesitated. "Sir, what I have is not fit for you." He was carrying a kind of country liquor, called *natadi*, commonly made from the palmyra tree.

"It doesn't matter; come on, give me some," he said, and he drank it. The students suddenly found that they were thirsty, too, so they also drank from the pot. The group began moving forward, with the disciples weaving here and there, drunk. They had walked a few miles more in the hot sun when Shankara said, "I'm thirsty again."

He noticed a shop at the side of the road where a blacksmith was boiling lead in a pot. The liquid was milky and white, so he said, "You seem to be boiling some milk." Without even giving the blacksmith a chance to say anything, he took some of the liquid and drank it. Then he looked at the disciples and said, "I think all of you must be thirsty; come, drink!" They immediately realized their mistake and fell at his feet. "Now we see; we cannot imitate you in everything."

If a small plant wants to imitate a big tree and says, "I don't want any fence around me. That big fellow doesn't have any fence," what will happen? The cows will come and eat it. We should know our limitations. Let us not simply say, "Jesus did it. Moses did it." Moses spoke to God. With whom do you speak?

I once went to visit the Christian monks on the Greek island of Mt. Athos. I was surprised to find them all strict vegetarians. It reminded me of the very first thing that the Bible says about diet: "And God said, 'Behold, I have given you every herb-bearing seed, which is upon the face of the earth, and every tree, in which are fruits; for you it shall be as meat.'"(Genesis 1:29) The *Dead Sea Scrolls* contain some of the teachings from the time of Jesus on meat-eating: "And the flesh of slain beasts in a person's body will become his own tomb. For I tell you truly, he who kills, kills himself, and whosoever eats the flesh of slain beasts eats the body of death." And when St. Paul went out preaching he said in his letter to the Romans, "It is good not to eat flesh . . ." (Romans 14:21).

I have also had the opportunity to read some of the works of the 14th Century Christian saints recorded in the library of manuscripts housed at the Order of the Cross in England. Almost every one recommended pure vegetarian food and no liquor, even in the name of Eucharist. Some of them even laughed at the people who ate meat and used wine in that way. They said, "If you people want to drink, don't bring God in there. Go home and drink, but don't bring it to the altar." Why? They said, "How can you expect your mind to be clean when you are taking meat and alcohol?"

That is the reason almost every religion advocates at least some days of adherence to vegetarian diet. Whether they know the reasons or not, religious people of many different faiths stay away from animal food on auspicious days. They call it an "Ash Wednesday," or a "Good Friday." Why is it a "Good Friday"? By not eating meat, you make it a good Friday, a holy day.

The Chinese celebrate their New Year's Day with strict vegetarian diet. New Year's is a new beginning and they want it to be very auspicious and holy, so they stay away from meat. By staying away from meat you make a day holy. If you stay away from meat every day, *every* day will be a holy day. Consciously or not, we recognize the effect of food on the mind and know that a vegetarian diet leaves the mind more serene, more peaceful.

Economic & Ecological Considerations

Our human family is starving in many parts of the world. People say that there isn't enough food for us all, that overpopulation is the cause. But I say that overpopulation is not the problem; rather, human greed is the problem. If we were only willing to care and share, there would be enough for everyone.

How can I say this? According to agricultural statistics, you must feed sixteen pounds of grain to a steer in order to get one pound of meat. The amount of grain we use to produce meat is almost equal to the amount consumed as food in the poorer countries.

Another way of looking at it is this: On the average, an acre of land used for grain production gives five times as much protein as an acre used for producing meat; an acre of beans or lentils gives ten times as much protein; and an acre of vegetables, fifteen times as much protein. So to feed a meat-eater, how much more land is needed! If everyone were to become a vegetarian, there would be plenty of food and plenty of protein for everyone. As Mahatma Gandhi used to say, "The earth has enough for everyone's need, but not enough for everyone's greed."

CHAPTER 5:
BECOMING A VEGETARIAN

Two Approaches

Many people ask, "How do I go about becoming a vegetarian?" One way is to make a gradual transition to vegetarian diet. Leave off eating red meat, but continue eating fish and fowl for some time. Then leave off the fowl, and eat only fish and eggs for some time. And then, finally, eat only vegetarian food. But if you are totally convinced of the value of becoming a vegetarian and you have strong willpower, I would recommend that you drop it all right away. When you discover that something is not good for you, why not reject it?

The body, which is used to the flesh food, may still "demand" it. You may feel a kind of addiction, like the craving for the nicotine in cigarettes. Your cells remember it; they still have the toxins in them. So it may be difficult at first. If your body is very much saturated with toxins, you may face some headaches, even some nausea, until the toxins are purged out. If it happens that way, it certainly is not going to kill you. And there are some things that will help you, should you find yourself experiencing any uneasiness.

To begin a transition to vegetarianism, I would recommend that you don't take any stimulants, such as coffee or tea, during this transition period. Why? Because the coffee brings caffeine—another kind of toxin—into your system. When the caffeine comes in, it invites its sister, purine, which is a toxin found in meat. Then those two call for their other sister, nicotine. I call them the I-N-E sisters. That's why, after a sumptuous meat dinner, you want a cup of coffee in one hand and a cigarette or cigar in the other. They all go together.

So at least for a while, try to stay away from stimulants such as coffee and tea. For anyone who might be trying to quit smoking, these things will also be helpful. Drink a lot of pure water. Take some saunas. Sunbathe if possible. Sweat a lot. All of these things will push out the toxins from your system and relieve the discomfort. When the toxins are gone, you will lose the craving for meat. Another way is simply to begin practicing the Yoga postures and breathing. I have seen many, many people who did not choose to become vegetarians consciously, but found that the habit of meat-eating fell away when they took up Yoga practice. The system becomes cleaner and more sensitive to the toxic effects of a meat diet.

Living With Non-Vegetarians

Often one member of a family will want to be a vegetarian while the others do not. You may even have to cook for meat-eating members of the family. What should you do? If they aren't yet ready to understand the importance and benefit of a vegetarian diet, you should accept that. If you are the one to cook and they want you to prepare meat, you can feel, "It's my duty to provide for them; it need not upset me." If you demand that they change, you are forcing your ideas on them. Instead, let them decide for themselves that they want to change by seeing the beauty of your life.

When they see you always healthy, happy, and peaceful, let them ask, "What is your secret?" You can just answer, "It's because of my diet." If they are sensible they will also slowly change. Meanwhile, just give them their food. There is nothing wrong in it. It will not make you a non-yogi or a violent person. On the other hand, it will make you a better yogi if you do it pleasantly, with a loving heart.

Sometimes there is a tendency to become arrogant. You might feel: "Oh, I am a big yogi now. I stopped eating meat, drinking, smoking. I am a holy person now, a pure person." You might find yourself putting others down. That is yogic arrogance. If you really want to be a good yogi, be more humble. Humility will bring out all of your beautiful qualities. That way you can help many people. Humility is the greatest virtue because it shows people that you have learned a lot, that you are rich in knowledge. Anything that is very light and hollow will rise up in a balance. Anything that is heavy will sink. Have you ever seen a wheat plant growing? As long as the wheat grains are raw, not yet rich with nutrition, they will stand upright, as if to say, "Here I am!" As they slowly become ripened, they become heavy and bend down. Likewise with us if we have rich, good qualities we will bow down. Don't hesitate to say to people, "I don't know." If they still demand to know your secret, you can say, "Well, because you are asking, I will tell you what I know, what I feel." Share what you have with humility.

Sometimes it's the person who does the cooking who insists that the others should eat meat, or that all the family members should eat the same thing at a meal. You can explain, "I am eating for my stomach and you are eating for yours. Although we are a family, we still have some personal things. Because we are one family, if I need to use the toilet, should you also come and sit on the toilet?" Or if another family member demands that the food you eat be the same, suggest, "Then why not the quantity also?" Another may eat one piece of toast; you may eat three pieces. Should he or she say, "We are one family; we should eat the same amount?" No; it doesn't make sense.

If the other one still insists, you can try a little acting. Say, "Okay, honey, to satisfy you I will eat what you want." Put it in your mouth, chew it, swallow it, and then pretend you are sick, that you are going to throw up. Just start rushing to the bathroom. Surely the loved one will say, "Oh, no, I can see that this food is not for you. I'm so sorry." That's better than just saying, "I'm not going to eat *that* —I'm a vegetarian, I'm pure!" That will just create bad feelings in the family.

Occasionally, a child might be the one who wants to eat meat in a vegetarian home. Here I would say that there are many things we do not allow children to decide for themselves until they grow to a certain maturity. Until then you have a duty to bring them up along the right lines, in a way conducive to their health. Children should have freedom, but in certain areas they do not yet know what is right and what is wrong. If a child doesn't know how to use a knife, will you put it in those inexperienced hands just because the child cries for it? No. You are the caretaker.

It's our duty as parents to do everything possible for the sake of the children. If it's you who still eats meat and you don't want to give it up, but you want your child to be a vegetarian, probably you should make the change, at least for the child's sake. The modern way is for parents to have a glass of whiskey in one hand, a cigarette in the other, and say, "Child, I never want to see you drinking or smoking!" If you absolutely cannot set an example, at least do these things out of their sight. Remember that children are not playthings. Raising children is a big responsibility. For that we may have to change ourselves too.

CHAPTER 6:

QUESTIONS & ANSWERS

Should Our Pets Be Vegetarians Too?

Dogs and cats are carnivores by nature. They can live on vegetarian food, but it's not their natural diet. Just because a vegetarian diet is recommended for us, that doesn't mean we should try to make everyone and everything else follow it too. Certainly the meat-eaters are not trying to feed their cows meat. Then why should we try to make the dogs and cats vegetarians? It will not be bad karma for you to feed them their meat because you aren't eating it. Your dog serves you as a watchdog or in other ways and you are taking care of it. If you have a car that runs on high octane gas, you buy high octane gas. If you have a diesel car, you should buy diesel fuel. So give your pets their own type of food; there is nothing wrong in it.

What Can We Do About Garden Pests?

Another question often asked is, "What about the insects that feed on the vegetables we are growing? Is it wrong to kill them?" You are growing the food for your use, not for theirs. If you want to be really kind to them, allot a small patch for them: "That is your area; you can eat all you want over there, but don't come here." If you feel you must forcefully remove them from your vegetables, warn them every day for three days. Each time make the warning stronger, and on the third day tell them, "This is your final warning. Those who do not leave are going to be destroyed." Then, if there are any left, you can do it. If you have given such a warning, your conscience will be clear. The insects will leave. The same principle applies to weeds; the life force will even depart from the weeds with such a warning. That is the most gentle way.

Is Vegetarianism Necessary for Attaining Enlightenment?

I am not recommending vegetarian diet because it is the only way to attain enlightenment. I advocate it because it helps you physically and mentally to make yourself more relaxed and calm, so that you can realize the spirit within sooner. It is a help, but it is not a must. If you have the capacity to control the mind, to keep it tranquil under all circumstances, you can certainly eat anything you want; you can lead any life you want. What is necessary is to keep the mind tranquil, because only in tranquility of mind can the God within you express itself, or be realized. And, generally, meat is a *rajasic* food that brings restlessness to the mind. If you have a strong mind you can probably win over that. There have certainly been saints who ate meat, but I would say that they are the exception, not the rule.

Many people tell me, "Well, I'm a vegetarian, *more or less*. Isn't it all right to eat a little fish or chicken every once in a while?" If you kill a chicken once in a while, it's still murder. If you eat it, you're still taking dead matter into your system, poisoning yourself. It's not that doing so will damage your life completely, but when you know these things, why should you do it even "once in a while?" In Hinduism they talk about certain vows, which are called the *maha vratam* or great vows. For these, there are almost no exceptions. If the act is wrong—like stealing or killing—it is wrong. There *can* be exceptions; for example, if your life is that important to the world, and if it could be saved only by killing a chicken, fine. But that isn't the same as going to a party and thinking, "Oh, I'll just eat a little; otherwise, what will they think?" If they will be that offended, act a little: "I am sorry, but my doctor asked me not to eat it because it doesn't seem to agree with me." Don't use their displeasure as an excuse for breaking your vow.

What About Eggs & Dairy Products?

Eggs partake of the same quality as flesh. This is even true of unfertilized eggs. How do we know this? When you break an egg and leave it, it rapidly begins to decay and give off a foul odor just as meat does. This is why vegetarians avoid eggs as well as meat.

Those who like not to use dairy are better vegetarians. I leave it to the individuals to decide. Strictly speaking we don't need dairy products. They are not necessary. No animal drinks milk when it is grown. The cow produces milk to be given to the calf. After some time the calf stops drinking. But humans continuously drink and consume too much of dairy products.

Milk products do have a different quality than meat. Some people will say, "Milk comes from the cow. If you are going to drink the milk, why not eat the flesh?" When you were a baby, you drank milk from your mother's breast, is it not? Will you then cut the flesh from your mama to eat too? It is not the same thing. Milk products don't have the concentrated fat that meat has. Unlike eggs, if you leave milk out, it will curdle or turn sour, but it will not give off the foul smell of decaying flesh. Of course, if you drink too much of it, or if you do not digest it well, it will cause mucus and phlegm. And certainly we can live very well without milk products, eating only fruits, vegetables, legumes, grains, and nuts.

PART II:

THE YOGA OF EATING

by Sri Swami Satchidananda

CHAPTER 7:

KNOWING WHAT,
WHEN & HOW TO EAT

We have considered the benefits of a vegetarian diet. Is there more to be said about yogic diet? Yes; because *what* we eat, *when* we eat, and *how* we eat are all important parts of Yoga. First of all, what do we mean by yogic diet? The purpose of all Yoga practice is to keep the mind tranquil under all circumstances. Only in that tranquility of mind will the spirit in you express itself. When the mind is tranquil you see the God in you. All of our Yoga disciplines are to help us maintain this peacefulness. Food also plays an important part.

First, let us look at the physical side. In Yoga we acknowledge that the body and mind are intimately connected and that achieving mental poise is much more difficult when the body is not strong and well. So having robust health is often considered a helpful step in yogic life. Here I would like to say that our food is the major cause of our physical illnesses. What we eat, we become. If we eat junk food, our bodies will have to be junked.

I hear people say, "I don't have time to worry about meals . . . I usually just grab something and run." If you just "grab something," be careful, because something else will probably grab you. We should know what we are eating. In fact, if you can't get the right food on a certain day, it would be better for you to fast for that day. We don't fall sick by not eating. As statistics show, people fall ill by overeating or by eating the wrong food, not by abstaining from food. We should take care of our food first. Let it be clean; let it give life to us. Let it contain real nutrition, not just mere taste. So a part of Yoga practice, then, is dietary management. Eat the right toxin-free diet, in the right quantity, and in the right way.

How Much Food?

We do not need the amount of food we sometimes think we do. People often ask me what my diet is like. I tell them that there is a continuous, relaxed state in my mind that transmits into my body also. There is no stress at all, so my body does not need much food. My fuel economy is very good. People waste a lot of energy in worrying. Our anxiety about the future drains a lot of energy. People who worry drain their batteries completely. They have to eat more. But in my case, I never drain my *prana*, my vital energy, so I can live on very little; I can even live on air alone.

Somehow we have come to think, "Oh, I have to eat a lot to have enough energy." No. If you don't waste your energy, you will need very little. You can even take that energy directly from the elements. Through food, we get the elements; but if we know how to take energy directly from the elements, we don't need other food at all. It is a well-known fact that in most of the Western countries people fall sick because they overeat. During World War II, there was a food shortage in many parts of Europe. At that time half of the hospitals were empty. People didn't eat as much and they did not fall sick.

So we have to understand our systems. How much energy have we used up in our activities? How much do we need to replenish? There is a very simple way to know. Ask your stomach before you eat: "Tummy, are you wanting more? Have you used up what I gave you earlier?" Unless the stomach says, "Yes, I am ready," we should not eat. Many people eat for the other two "t's": "time" and the "tongue." They say, "Oh, it's 12 o'clock, I must have my lunch." Or, "What delicious pie, I must finish it." Instead, look to the third "t," the tummy. There's a beautiful saying in one of the works by the South Indian saint Thiruvalluvar which says, "The body will never need medicine if food is never taken without making sure that the stomach has digested what was given to it before."

Hunger is the sign for that. Hunger is the only reliable clock for when you should eat.

Here, too, we should know what true hunger is. If your hunger "pangs" go away within a short time, then what you felt was not true hunger at all. Such hunger pangs are based on habitual eating patterns, which create a sense of false hunger. They will go away roughly within half an hour. True hunger will not go away until you have eaten something.

Digestive Fire

I believe that proper digestive fire is much more important than a so-called balanced diet. The system knows how to balance itself. If we have that digestive fire burning within, and if we sometimes eat the wrong food, we will be able to digest it. Our digestive capacity is very important. Anything left undigested in the stomach will ferment and become acid, which gives us gas. So we should eat only when we are really hungry, and just to the limit. Then we can digest anything and everything.

If your digestion is a little weak, then you have to look for foods that have less of a mucus-producing tendency. In this regard, meat is the worst. You have to cook meat for a long time, and it takes a lot of energy to digest. It is very concentrated. Dairy products are often thought to be especially mucus-producing, and that is true, especially if your system is weak.

But even among the vegetables and fruits, some are more mucus-producing than others. These are the foods with more water content, cucumber or melon, for example. Because they cool the system, the digestive fire is immediately lowered when you eat them. Starchy foods, such as root vegetables, also take more fire to digest. The stomach is like a big oven. If you put dry sticks in it, it burns well. If you put in raw green sticks, the fire goes down.

If you put a banana peel on the fire it goes down even more. So remember to eat according to the hunger and according to the fire in the stomach.

Here again, we should remember that every fireplace is different. Not all of us have the same amount of fire. The label on something may say, "This is good food; this contains so much protein," but you might not be able to digest that much. Often we see charts that say, "If you weigh this much and your height is such and such, you should eat so many calories and so much protein." But nobody looks at the stomach inside: how big it is, how much fire it has, how sluggish it is. We need to prescribe a diet for our stomachs, not for the height and weight of our bodies.

When we eat in relation to when we expend energy is also very important. We should finish eating at least two hours before sleeping, and the evening food should be light. If you go to bed with undigested food in the stomach, some of your energy will go into digesting and you will not get a very good rest. The mid-day meal could be heavier because you will have plenty of time to digest, and you will be using the energy you get from that food later on. But first it is best to rest quietly for a while after a heavy meal.

Taking time for digestion is very important. In India we have a saying, "When the stomach is full, the brain is dull." After eating heavy food you yawn, you cannot think well. This is because you need circulation in the brain to think and the circulation has gone down to the stomach. If you force the blood to come to the brain, then the stomach will suffer. If your work does not allow you time to rest after lunch, then have a lighter lunch and an earlier dinner.

The biggest surprise for many people who are learning about yogic diet is the yogic approach to breakfast. People often think that having a big meal first thing in the morning is important because they will need the energy for their work. On the contrary, when we first wake up, the digestive fire is not that strong; it is still partly sleeping. So the morning food should be light.

There is a yogic saying that if you eat once a day you are a yogi; twice a day, you are a *bhogi*, and three times a day, a *rogi*. What does it mean? A yogi is a spiritual, well-balanced person. *Bhoga* means enjoyment, so if you want to just enjoy the world, eat twice a day. And *roga* means sickness; if you eat three times a day, you will probably fall sick very often.

The Nine-Gated City

We want to keep our bodies clean and problem-free. In order to accomplish this, we need to check what goes into them. If you want to keep a country in good shape, you establish check points—immigration entry points—at all of your borders. People must show their passports and visas before you let them in. We want to know, "Are you a good person or a criminal?" And if someone brings fruit into the country, "Is it healthy fruit or has it been bitten by insects?" Why? Because you want to preserve the health of the country. In the same way, your body is the place in which you live.

In Sanskrit it is called *navadwara puri* or the "nine-gated city." It has nine major gates and millions of minor gates, such as the skin pores. Imagine that you are thirsty and want to drink some water. First, two inspectors come to check it out: the eyes. "Well, it looks clean." Then another inspector comes on the job: the nose. "Smells fine." Then the third inspector, the mouth. "Yes, it tastes okay; let it pass through."

What kind of diet will keep us healthy then? One that is plain and simple that will keep the mind calm and serene and the body relaxed and free from toxins. It should agree with your system. It should be easy to digest. It should require a minimum amount of time to prepare. And it should be easy to clean up after. That is the basic guideline.

Still people ask, "But can't you tell us *exactly* what to eat?" No. Don't we say, "One person's nectar is another person's poison?" Each one has to decide what is right for him or her to eat. Books may be able to give you some guidance, but ultimately you are the one who must determine what is good for you. How? By paying attention to your body. Observe your stomach. Watch its reaction to a particular food and see how it agrees with you. If it does not agree, stay away from that, or lessen the quantity. Become your own dietician. This is an important part of Yoga. You need to see what you can digest well without producing mucus or gas. Those are symptoms of indigestion. If you feel a little stuffed up or puffy, it means that you either ate the wrong food or ate the wrong quantity of food—something beyond your capacity to digest.

Solid, Liquid, Gas

The type of activities in which you engage are very important in determining what you should eat. This idea is almost unrecognized in Western society. The proportion of solids and liquids in your diet should go hand in hand with the type of work you do. The more physical labor you do, the more solid food you should take. If you do more mental work, you can take more liquid food and not so much solid food. A person doing hard manual labor might need three meals of solid food a day; whereas a desk worker who is mostly sitting and thinking should not eat more than one solid meal a day to keep in good health.

People who are mostly meditating, or doing things with complete ease, can take more energy from the air itself. From solid, to liquid, to gas: If the need is for physical energy we take food from a solid source; if the need is mental, from liquid; and if the need is spiritual, then from a gaseous source. Children who are growing need quite a lot of physical energy to make their bodies grow well, so they could eat solid food quite often.

Make Changes Slowly

We must decide what is best for our systems, but we do not need to be fanatics. Go slowly. Maybe you have decided that white bread is not good for you, that it is made from white flour, which is good for gluing up posters and will glue up your intestines as well. In that case, if you can buy whole grain bread, fine, do it. But if you go home and immediately toss out all the white flour products in your home, your family might go wild. Instead, know the direction in which you want to go and then proceed slowly, gently. Poison is poison, whether it is a little or a lot; but some poisons will kill you immediately, while others harm you more slowly. Think of where you are, who you are with and your capacity—and then use your common sense.

Suppose you go to the home of a good friend or a relative and you are served white bread or something similar made with all love for you. You need not immediately say, "Hey, I'm a Yogi; I can't eat this rubbish!" The harm to your friend's feelings is worse than the harm the bread would do to you. Take a taste; act as if you are really enjoying it, and eat more of the vegetables. You have to judge what is more important in a situation. But, if you are really keen in improving your diet, there is always a way. If you want to avoid caffeine, but you still want a hot drink like coffee, you can take one of the many caffeine-free beverages: grain coffees, coffee substitutes, and herbal teas. Anywhere there is a will, there is a way.

How to Eat

How we eat our food is also very important. Do not use your mouth as a funnel to get the food to the stomach as quickly as possible! How often we see people shovel it in and the next minute it is gone. We should be using all of our 32 teeth to chew, and we should be chewing well. As I mentioned before, digestion actually begins in the mouth; there are digestive enzymes in the saliva itself. The saying, "Well begun is half done," can be applied to the digestion also.

I would also recommend that you take care to eat at a time when your body and mind are well relaxed. If you are upset, angry, or agitated for any reason, it's better not to eat at that time. You will literally be poisoning your system. It's also better not to prepare food for yourself or for others at such a time, because those vibrations will go into the food you are cooking and affect those who eat it.

It is best to prepare food with a calm mind, and to sit silently for a few moments before you begin eating, taking some time to consciously relax the body and let go of any distracting or disturbing thoughts in the mind. A short prayer of dedication or thanksgiving (see page 81) might be said during this time, or you might just want to spend a moment in silent meditation.

Generally, I would suggest that you take your meals in silence. It's best to concentrate on the food while you are eating it. You will digest better and enjoy your meal more. How many times do we get so engrossed in conversation that we don't even taste the food? If there is conversation, it should be light and pleasant.

A "business" lunch or dinner does not do justice to either the business or the meal. The business deal will be sounder if your mind is only on the business and if part of your energy is not going into digestion. And your stomach will be happier if you focus all of your attention on your food while you are eating. This kind of awareness will also help a lot if you tend to have a problem with eating more than you should.

CHAPTER 8:
THE PROPERTIES OF FOOD

In yogic thinking, everything in nature is divided into three groups according to the three *gunas* or qualities mentioned before: *sattva*, *rajas*, and *tamas*. *Sattva* is the tranquil state, *rajas* the very active state, and *tamas* the state of inertia or dullness. One of the main scriptures of Yoga, the *Bhagavad Gita*, speaks at great length on the qualities of different diets. Foods that are close to their natural state—not very spicy, sour, or hot—are considered to be *sattvic*. These include fruits, nuts, vegetables (raw and cooked), cooked grains, and peas, lentils, or beans.

When the same products are mixed with a lot of spices and become sour or hot, they become *rajasic*. That means they create a restlessness in the mind. Since our main goal is to keep the mind in a tranquil state, we use the aid of everything in our daily lives to retain a state of health and tranquility. *Rajasic* food also includes meat and other flesh food. They make us active in a restless, sometimes aggressive, way. All foods that are old, overcooked, or very cold, come under the *tamasic* category. That would also include any food that has been cooked and then kept for a long time or food that is moldy.

The manner in which we eat can also make the resulting state of body and mind *sattvic*, *rajasic*, or *tamasic*. For example, if we do not chew a *sattvic* food well, so that it can be well assimilated, it will ferment within the body and can cause *tamas* or the quality of inertia. Or, if we overeat or eat right before going to sleep, we will also become *tamasic*.

According to Ayurveda, the ancient Indian system of medicine, foods can also be divided according to the effect they have on the body. The categories are: *vata* or wind-producing; *pitta* or bile, producing; and *kapha*, mucus-producing. All foods and herbs can be categorized that way. Some of each quality will be found in every food, but one of the three qualities will be predominant.

Take, for example, the mucus-producing category: all pumpkins and gourds have a lot of water, and so they are cooling and produce mucus. However, this does not mean that they are not good food. If your body produces more bile, you may need exactly those foods to counteract the bile and bring a balance. Or you might need to take a food like eggplant, which is wind-producing. In Ayurveda, you are helped to maintain a balance by taking foods of the categories other than the one that is predominant in you.

This philosophy goes even deeper. The wind-producing food is associated with the element air, the bile-producing with fire, and the mucus-producing with water. Everything in nature comes from the five elements. Moreover, each element comes from the one before it—from ether, comes air; from air, comes fire; from fire, comes water; and from water, comes earth. That is why I say you can convert any one food into all the elements you need for health if your system is pure, strong, and subtle. There are people—mostly great saints and sages—who are able to live on air alone. You can experiment a little with this yourself. If you practice a lot of *pranayama*—the yogic breathing—your physical food consumption will go down. You will not feel the need to eat as much because you will be getting your nourishment from the *prana* itself.

Food Combining

The idea of a mono-diet is often used in the naturopathic approach to healing. Mono-diet means eating only one thing at a time, rather than putting a lot of different foods into the stomach at the same time: one type of fruit, or one vegetable, or one grain, for example. If you eat this way, your body will digest the food more easily and assimilate it much better.

Therefore, I suggest that if you want to eat some fruit, eat just one kind of fruit at a time. Eat one—or even four—apples, but do not mix them with cantaloupe. If you are eating carrots, eat only carrots for that meal. Your stomach will be grateful to you because it will have just one thing to do; digestion will be much quicker and easier. This is because each food takes a different amount of time to digest and utilizes different enzymes.

Digestion is similar to cooking in this way. When you want to make a vegetable stew, you do not put everything into the pot at once. You put the roots first, later the broccoli, and much later, the leafy green vegetables. So think of the stomach as a cooking pot. Sometimes I have seen people eating steamed vegetables with fried food. The fried things will take a longer time to digest, whereas the steamed vegetables take much less time.

If you really feel you need a little more variety, then eat two or three things together that would be digested in a similar way and in the same amount of time. For instance, it is especially helpful not to have cooked and raw food at the same meal. And as a general rule, I would advise that if you are eating solid food, you should stick to solids; if you are drinking, have only liquids.

This idea, too, is almost unknown in the West. We often see people drinking coffee or wine while eating meat and vegetables, or ending a meal with a beverage. Even water should not be taken during a meal of solids. It will dilute the digestive juices. Liquids should be taken an hour or two before or after solid food. If you get thirsty while you are eating, it is because you are not chewing enough before swallowing. If you chew well, you will not feel thirsty. I often say that you should drink your solids and eat your liquids. How? When eating, chew the food well until the solids break down and become a liquid, mixing completely with your saliva. When drinking, mix the liquids well in your mouth and swallow them slowly, as you do when you chew.

Another bad habit many people have is drinking milk with other food. Perhaps if you really want something else, you could have a banana with it. Often we see people eating or drinking citrus at the same time as milk. It sounds like common sense to say these should never be combined; no one would pour orange juice into a glass of milk. But think how common it is for people to have a breakfast that includes orange juice in a glass and milk in a bowl of cereal. We should think of how all these principles might be applied.

Today there is also a lot of concern about how to get enough fiber in one's diet. Food that is eaten whole and raw has a lot of fiber in it. For example, when you eat a whole raw apple you get fiber from the cellulose coating. Almost everything should be eaten with the husk on it: vegetables, fruits, beans, even grains. We spend money to take the bran out of the wheat for white flour products; then we spend money to buy extra bran to supplement our diet. If we eat products in their whole state, we will get plenty of fiber.

There is another advantage to eating raw food. We consume much less of the same food when it is not cooked. Take cauliflower, for example. The average person could not eat even half of a raw cauliflower. But if it were cooked, the same person could easily eat the entire vegetable. By eating uncooked food, we save food, we get more fiber, and at the same time we save time and energy in preparing it. I often say that the day human beings learned to cook their food was the day they began laying the foundations for the hospitals.

Food & Pain

When we overeat or eat the wrong thing, we may experience a stomachache, headache, pain, or nausea and vomiting. If you put toxins into the system, they will accumulate and cause you pain. Why? They are saying, "Somehow you accumulated us. We won't be helpful to you, so please get us out of here and remember not to put any more in." If it were not for the headache, you would torture the body more and more. Without the stomach pain, you would keep on gobbling. It is the physical pain that brings us this message. The body is telling you, "I have had enough; you are torturing me too much. Stop it." The pain itself is an alarm, a warning.

But what do we often do? We kill the pain that brings the message. First you put in all the steak, hot dogs, beer, and junk food. Then the body cries out: "My God, I am not made for this. I am a simple thing. I just want simple, plain vegetables. Why are you putting all this junk into me? I cannot take it anymore." Instead of listening, we say, "How dare you tell me that? If you continue to give me this message, not only will I keep on eating as I please, but I am going to destroy you with a pain killer." It is as if the fire alarm in your home goes off and you wake up and say, "Hey, you miserable alarm!," and then get up, cut the wire, and go back to sleep. Would you do that? No. You would get up and find out what was setting off the alarm. Likewise, we should be looking for the cause of our pain.

CHAPTER 9:

FASTING

Fasting is a natural process. Animals do it. Almost every spiritual and folk tradition in the world talks about it. It is only in recent times that people seem to have come to fear it and to feel that they must eat every day no matter what. The body is like any other factory. You make the machines work all week, then you give them some down time for rest or cleaning and overhauling. In the same way, even if we are eating the right food, our digestive systems need a little rest from their ordinary routine. Actually, it is more like a "break" than a rest, because the system takes advantage of that time to burn up any toxins or excess fat that might have been inadvertently put into it. It overhauls itself and gets ready for the next day's work.

If we eat the proper foods and have only a light supper, our system has a mini-fast every night during which it gets cleaned up and the stomach gets some rest. Unfortunately, our heavy dinners and late evening meals often prevent that, and longer fasts of a day or more become advisable at such times. For a healthy person with a reasonably good diet, I recommend one day of fasting a week. It can be any day that is convenient for you, but stick to the same day each week—perhaps a weekend day so that you can have more quiet time. This will take care of any small problems in your system before they can become big problems.

If fasting is good for healthy people, it is even more important for those who are weak or sick. When your body is sick, your stomach is also sick. By eating, you make your sick stomach work more. Instead, allow it to rest and heal. There is a saying in Sanskrit, the translation is: "Fasting is the best medicine." Normally, when you are ill, you do not feel much like eating. So it is more natural not to eat at such times. If you want to help cure almost any ailment, stay away from food until you feel the symptoms subside and experience real hunger again. When you give that rest to your system, your vital energy inside will act as an inner doctor to burn up the toxins that have created the sickness. This applies also to any extra fat or toxins, minor physical problems, and aches and pains in the body. When you fast, you eliminate the toxins, digest the undigested food, assimilate the extra fat, and come back to normal health.

The following are some general guidelines on fasting. If you have any doubts or questions on undertaking a fast for yourself, it would be best to consult an expert in the field.

What to Take During Your Fast

In my experience, the best way to fast is to just drink plain water. On certain religious holidays, some people even fast without water. In India, when devotees fast without water and they feel thirsty, they put a few peppercorns in their mouths, bite them gently, and when the saliva comes, they swallow it. But if you are fasting for health reasons, I would recommend drinking plenty of water. If that is too difficult for you, then take juice diluted with water. I hear of people drinking carrot juice four or five times a day on their fast. Each glass of carrot juice takes six or seven carrots to make, so in a day you might be consuming thirty or forty raw carrots in the form of juice. I would not recommend this. One should take diluted fruit juices, such as grape or orange juice, that are more watery. Watermelon is also excellent to have while fasting.

Enemas & Purgatives

It is good to take enemas regularly once or even twice a day while you are fasting. This is because the system gets heated when you fast; even the colon develops heat. Since the moisture from the waste matter will then be absorbed back into the system, it is better to eliminate the waste. Even before beginning the fast, you might want to take a purgative to clean the bowels. I would recommend castor oil or another natural type of purgative. This is especially important if you are fasting to cure an infection. Any inflammation in the body will be aggravated, and any swelling will become more painful, if the stomach or colon is still heavy with the undigested, fermented matter.

Symptoms of Cleansing

You should know in advance that you may experience some unpleasant symptoms while fasting. If you know that they are all signs of cleansing, you will welcome them and not become frightened. The symptoms come because toxins are being removed from the organs, glands, and tissues into the bloodstream, and are then being eliminated through the perspiration, breath, urine, and solid wastes. It is similar to cleaning a carpet in your home. Before you disturb the carpet, the house might look beautiful and clean. But the minute you start moving and shaking the rug, all kinds of dust and dirt come out.

The same thing happens while fasting; all the toxins come out. You may experience a headache because of it. If so, drink more water. If you feel nauseated, drink a lot of water and then throw it right up. I have heard people say, "Oh, whenever I stop eating I get nauseated, I get a headache. So I must eat." That is incorrect. These are signs that you are cleaning out the body. If you stick with it, the headache and nausea will go away.

Sometimes you will suddenly feel that you have lost all your strength. That is fine. Do not do anything strenuous for a while, but continue the fast. The tongue will get coated, and your breath and saliva may smell and taste foul. That is because the whole "rug" is being shaken and all the dirt is being tossed up.

I recommend that you sunbathe if possible during your fast so that you will perspire and cleanse more. Sunbathing is like a very mild sauna that does not stress the system. Deep breathing is also an excellent way to help eliminate the toxic material more quickly. The Yoga *kriyas* are also good: especially nasal cleansing with water (using a *neti* pot) and the stomach wash.

How Long to Fast

How long you should fast depends on how much toxic material you have accumulated in your system. It might take two days to eliminate, or four, or ten. There are very definite signs that let you know when you have finished, however. You will feel light. Your saliva will become clean, clear, and sweet-tasting, like spring water. Your tongue will no longer be coated. Your eyesight will be sharper. All of the senses will become more alert, and you will not have any feeling of dullness or drowsiness. An amazing feeling of strength will come. You may not have the strength to do physical work, but you will feel like running, like flying!

At one time I was living at a place of pilgrimage in South India where the shrine is located one thousand steps up, at the very top of a hill. I fasted for a number of days, and after the fourth day I felt as if I could fly up the hill. When you get these signs, you know that it is time to break the fast. At that point you will feel a hunger that will not go away until you eat something. That is the time to break the fast.

How to Break a Fast

How you break a fast—and with what—is very important. I would even say that the way in which you break a fast is more important than the fast itself. If you fast for a few days, it is best to take the same amount of time to completely return to your normal diet. For example, if you fast for four days, take four days to break the fast, starting with lighter foods in small quantities. If your fast is longer, the same basic principle applies: take some time to gradually work up to eating denser foods and larger quantities again.

Here are some general guidelines: first have a liquid, such as diluted juice, if you have been fasting on water alone. The next step would be to have some coconut yogurt or probiotic capsules. You can cut up some pieces of cucumber, and some fresh coriander leaves if you can get them, and add this to the yogurt. For the next stage you might have something more solid, perhaps a light cooked cereal such as cooked brown rice cereal or cooked quinoa. Then progress to steamed vegetables. As you come out of the fast, slowly, slowly increase the density of your food until you are back to your normal diet. Never break a fast with a big meal or heavy food.

Often people can fast easily, but when the time comes to break the fast, they feel compelled to pounce on any and all food that comes within reach. This is where you will need strict control over the tongue. If you cannot control the tongue, it is better not to fast. Why? Because fasting is a reconditioning of the body. Every part of the system will become more delicate, more sensitive.

It is similar to overhauling an automobile engine. After an engine has been rebuilt, there is a breaking-in period: in first gear you should go only ten miles an hour; in second gear, only twenty miles an hour; in third gear, only forty miles an hour—for at least the first thousand miles. The engine must get used to working again. When you have reconditioned the body by fasting, you cannot run it at breakneck speed the following day. I see many people who fast for ten days, eat anything for two months, then fast for another ten days. This is very unhealthy for the body, and for the mind as well. If you cannot break your fast carefully, it is much better not to fast at all.

Fasting & the Mind

There is a higher significance to fasting also. Fasting helps to calm the mind. Mastering the body and senses will lead you to mastery of the mind. The body and senses themselves are never unruly. They are simply instruments. It is the mind that drives the senses. When the mind is not connected to the senses—in sleep, for example—they do not do anything. Even when you are awake, it often happens that you do not hear people when they call you because you are deeply engrossed in something. Why? The ears are always open, but in this case your mind is somewhere else.

The senses are all gateways to the mind, instruments through which the mind functions to experience things. When you gain mastery over the senses, such as the tongue in this case, you are indirectly gaining mastery over the mind. As mentioned before, that is one of the reasons that fasting is so often associated with spiritual and religious observances. So if you would like to have more control over your mind, fasting can help you to achieve it.

CHAPTER 10:

EATING TO LIVE
OR LIVING TO EAT?

Compulsive Eating

Many people suffer from the compulsion to overeat and seek to develop the willpower to overcome this problem. Developing such willpower is the entire purpose behind all of the Yoga practices. We want to have the control to use our will in the way we want. The best way to develop such will is to apply it to smaller things first. Start with something you feel you could easily accomplish. If you take something that is a big problem for you and immediately try to develop willpower in that area, you may fall down and lose your confidence. It can put more negativity into the mind and drain the will. That is because you are taking on a task beyond your present capacity.

In order to understand how to train the will, we should look at how a fitness trainer works with someone new to lifting weights. Before the person is expected to lift at their highest level, they are trained to always begin with a warm up and to begin with lighter weights. Over time, larger weights will be added next; then a little more weight. The idea is for the trainer to gradually increase the weight. That way the person gains confidence. "Oh, is that all? I can certainly do that." While the person is in such a confident and cooperative mood, he or she will barely even notice if a little more weight is added.

Our minds are also like that. A positive feeling, or self-confidence, is what you call "will." It is not something you have to—or even can—go and get from somewhere outside of you. Apply it little by little, always at a level where you feel positive and confident. For example, say you want to go on a fast. Before you overdo and fast for one whole week, just say, "Okay, for one day I am going to miss my lunch." You might think, "Oh, that's easy; anybody can do that!" Fine, do it. Then a week or two later, maybe go for a whole day with just a few glasses of juice. If you have confidence in doing that, then a week later, take just as many cups of water as you want for one day, but no juice. Keep up the confidence in yourself. This is the most important thing.

What I say may be enough advice for some people. But if you cannot change by yourself, you may need outside help to do it. Never feel that you *must* do it all by yourself. If it seems too much for you to do alone, seek the help of others.

Weight Gain

If you are one of the many people who worry a lot about being overweight, know that the worry itself will make you overweight. A heavy mind will make the body heavy. If you make your mind heavier due to anxiety about being overweight, your body will become heavier still. Most people eat more when they worry. The more you think of weight, the more you will create weight, one way or another. As you think, so you become. If you keep on saying, "I overeat; I must not overeat. I overeat; I must not overeat," you will certainly overeat. The best thing for you to do is to forget about it; then you will not do it. So to start with, even if the body is on the heavy side, keep the mind light. That is the first thing. Without the worry, you might even be able to make some healthy changes in your diet.

A lot of benefit could come from doing the Yoga practices regularly—the postures, the breathing, and the cleansing practices, or *kriyas*. Especially helpful would be *agnisara* (the fire breath), *nauli* (stomach churning), and *bhastrika* (the bellows breathing).

Sarvangasana (the shoulder stand) and *matsyasana* (the fish pose) will also help a lot in bringing balance to the thyroid gland, which regulates the metabolism. If you become adept at these practices, whatever you eat will be completely digested. There will not be any fat accumulating in the body. All of the practices in general will help a lot, especially if there is some sort of deficiency in the glands. The whole body can be affected if the glands are weak. If you rebuild the glands, the entire system will not get shaken by a problem in one area.

Individual Constitutions

If you are heavyset by nature, and believe that you must be thin, then you are buying the brainwashing of the business and advertising people. All kinds of things are sold to reduce your weight. Who says that you should weigh only so much? Each body is different. A horse is a horse; a deer is a deer. Both are very beautiful. Should one wish to be the other? Human constitutions also vary. Your make-up depends on who your father is, who your mother is, what your mother ate, what kind of elements she attracted to build up your body. If anyone is going to refuse your love because you weigh a few pounds more than some of the models in the magazines, then you should say goodbye to that person. As long as you are healthy, you should not worry. In fact, if you are constitutionally heavy and you starve yourself in order to reduce your weight, you will only weaken your health.

I come across many women in this situation. They feel that in order to be in style or to be popular, they must be slim or even skinny and bony. It has become the fashion that unless you are slim, you are not attractive and others will not even want to look at you. The first thing I would tell anyone caught in this trap is to shed this unhealthy notion. If a person is going to look at your flesh and bones, he or she must certainly be a butcher.

Only butchers are interested in flesh, bone and skin. The minute butchers see an animal, they mentally weigh it: *how much flesh can I get, what kind of nice hide can I get?* If a man or woman does not want to look at you, shun him or her. They are butchers then. They are interested only in your flesh. They are not interested in your qualities. The body is simply a vehicle. It can be long and sleek, or it can be round and compact. It can even be "ugly"—with some dents and scratches, or a missing fender—and still take you farther than some of the shiny new cars just coming off the assembly line.

Of course, we all know that underneath, the so-called beauties can be as ugly as scorpions and as poisonous as snakes. A cobra appears to be very beautiful—shiny, slim, and dancing—but there is a deadly poison within. Therefore, let us learn to look beyond the external beauty and appreciate the real beauty that lies within. Everyone would agree with this; but do we practice it? These are not new ideas. They are repeated over and over again. A well-known saint of South India named Avvaiyar presents this idea beautifully. She says that the hair, dress, and face powder will not really make a person beautiful. What will? The wisdom that dawns through your tranquility of mind. She is talking about Yoga. Yogic beauty is the real beauty, she says. It lies in the heart. People should learn to look at the beauty of the heart and mind first. Anyway, who says a heavy person is ugly? If God hated big bodies, certainly it would have been no trouble to make them all slim.

Weight Maintenance

If you *are* overweight, here is a practical hint for reaching and maintaining the weight that is proper for your constitution. You do not need to purposely reduce the quantity of food you eat. It will automatically be reduced if you just chew your food well. Chew it until it becomes liquefied in your mouth. You will find that half the amount you were eating before will now be enough. And, if possible, eat more leafy green vegetables.

If the habits are not too ingrained, another way to work on this compulsion is to analyze and train the mind. Ask the mind, "What are you gaining by overeating? Can't you see that you are not going to solve your problems this way? You are hiding from them behind the food. And not only that, in addition you are adding more problems.

If the mind does not want to cooperate, there is another way for it to learn. Relax and let yourself eat as much as possible. Simply eat as much as you can. Eat more and more. Give yourself full permission to do this. Eat until you feel you will burst. Eat until you get completely disgusted with it. If it is just one food that you eat compulsively, do this with that one food—ice cream, or bread, or whatever it is. You will reach a point where the mind will say, "I cannot touch it anymore." So either discuss the problem with your mind and convince it to change, or allow it to get so thoroughly disgusted that it is willing to change on its own.

As a final point, I would remind you that though we use the term "overeating," you can never really overeat. If you did "overeat," you would throw up immediately. The stomach would take care of it. Usually we overestimate our eating out of anxiety. Even if you eat very little on a given day, you may still worry that you are overeating. So know that the problem here is in the mind, and that the solution is in the mind also. Change the mind first, and a change in the body will follow.

Substance Addiction

We become addicted to substances that stimulate our systems. Overly spicy food, coffee, tea, alcohol, and drugs all seem to stimulate us, even though some of them may technically be called depressants. All of these may pick us up for a while; but later on we drop down to a level even lower than the one at which we started. With continued usage, our systems become weaker and weaker and we become more and more addicted to the substances to pick us up again. At first, one sip of beer would have pepped you up for a whole day; then slowly one bottle is needed, then two bottles, then a case. It is because the body becomes weaker, and you need a stronger dose. The same is true of sleeping pills and tranquilizers. With time, you need more and more to achieve the same effect.

If we want to get out of these addictions, we have to strengthen the body and mind. Some of these substances may appear to strengthen us, but they do not. Many people believe that these substances help them to think. When they get into some problem or when they are searching for an idea, and the solution does not come, they pick up their cigarettes or their cocaine. Immediately they think, "Ah, I got it!" That is because the stimulant accelerates the body and mind—but only for a while. Then it drops them down again.

There are some rock singers who roar at the top of their lungs. Where do they get the energy? From drugs. But if you see them afterwards, they are like wounded animals; you cannot even go near them. I know many of them. That is not real energy or real strength. Strength can only come from proper health, not from external things brought into the body.

You may say, "Yes, we know these things are bad for our health, but we have gotten used to them; we are addicted, how can we get out of it?" Here Yoga will help a lot. If a person practices Hatha Yoga—the Yoga postures and breathing—he or she can eliminate all the toxins from his or her body. Once the toxins are gone, the craving will be gone too. For example, someone who smokes a lot may realize that smoking is harmful and want to quit; but the craving is still there. It is as if there were two people in one body. There is the person who does not want to smoke anymore, and the one that does. Who is that "other person" who has the craving? It is the body that is already filled with nicotine. In other words, the nicotine that has already gone into you wants more nicotine. That is what you call craving.

If you want to get rid of these cravings, you need to push out the addictive substances—the toxins—that are already in you. This applies to any craving, any addiction: smoking, drinking, overeating, drugs. Simply start practicing Hatha Yoga and very soon you will see the craving getting weaker and weaker, eventually going away by itself. There are hundreds of proofs of this among my students. What happens is that the postures apply a gentle pressure in all the different areas of the body where the toxins are lodged, releasing them. As you come out of the postures, the pressure is relieved and the released toxins go into the bloodstream and get eliminated through the breath. The pressure also tones and strengthens the endocrine glands and nerve centers. The Yoga postures and breathing offer the best way to eliminate toxins.

CHAPTER 11:
DIET & HEALING

Put Healing on Speed Dial

If you have had an injury, an illness, or surgery, you should be especially careful to take only clean, simple, toxin-free food. Avoid coffee, tea, or other stimulants. If you do this, and relax well, you will be healed very quickly. I know of many, many instances of this. Here are a few examples.

Some time ago, when I was still living at my Guru's ashram in India, a woman who used to come there found out that she needed to have surgery to remove a large tumor. She asked me to oversee her convalescence. After the operation, she went to a relaxed place in the mountains with a nurse to attend to her. She ate only very clean, simple food and, although the nurse did not even want her to get up for a month, I soon had her walking daily in the fresh air. After ten days, she started doing Yoga postures. To her doctors' amazement, she was completely healed within one month.

Another notable case was that of my maternal uncle. He was always very strict with his diet, and never took coffee or tea. He was once in a very bad automobile accident, during which he received a large puncture wound in the head. The doctors at the hospital did what they could, and told him that he was not to go out for at least a month, until the wound was healed. To their surprise his head was completely healed within ten days. Not only was he a strict vegetarian, but he had never taken alcohol, coffee, or even tea in all of his life. In such cases, healing is many times faster than when the body is burdened with toxins.

Here is one more example. Once a radio announcer who was looking for a cure for his many allergies told me: "I am allergic to almost everything. The doctor told me not to eat this, not to touch that. And he gave me all of these pills. I don't know what to do. What do you think?" I said, "Add one more allergy to your list: pill allergy." He was worried about what would happen to him if he stopped taking all the pills. I told him, "Nothing will happen to you if you just follow a proper yogic diet." I also had him do some yogic breathing. He was quite heavy, so I did not even ask him to do the Yoga postures, just the breathing. Within ten days he was a thoroughly changed person. So you do not need to be allergic. Instead, take care not to fill your body with toxic material. Build up its natural strength. The allergies will disappear. They will become allergic to you!

Vitamins

I am often asked for my thoughts about taking vitamins. Taking the vitamins we need directly from the foods we eat is much better and more natural than taking them in the form of pills. But if the food you eat itself lacks the vitamins it should have because of the conditions under which it was grown, then there is no harm in supplementing your diet. You should not take too many however. When we consume large quantities of vitamins, we are mostly consuming money. The body can assimilate only so much of a vitamin, and what it cannot assimilate gets eliminated.

A lot of the benefit can be psychological too. For a long time doctors were saying, "Vitamin C cures colds." Many, many people thought that it was curing their colds. Now it is said, "Vitamin C does not cure colds." So it can be your own feeling of "Ah, I took Vitamin C; now I will be well!" that cures you.

CHAPTER 12:

SIMPLE REMEDIES

I was trained in homeopathy and nature cure, and practiced homeopathy when I was in Sri Lanka. I am often asked whether yogic diet can help with various simple health problems, and many people have had very good results from the suggestions I have given. By experimenting, you can learn to take care of many of your own ailments. Of course, in acute cases, it is always good to trust your doctor and his or her treatment. But for more simple problems, here are a few remedies. If you are interested, you can learn many more from naturopathic doctors and other natural health practitioners.

Sore Throat Remedy

If the sore throat was caused by excessive use of your vocal cords, there is probably inflammation, and you must stop using them as much as possible. Give the inflammation time to heal. If, on the other hand, it is due to some kind of mucus problem, such as most so-called colds and congestion, then you can take a mucus-free diet as a remedy. To help relieve the soreness while it is healing, make a paste out of honey (for vegans: substitute cardamom and/or vanilla-sweetened stevia plus licorice root) and ordinary ground black pepper, mixing them in whatever proportion you like. If it is too hot, use more honey; if it tastes too sweet, put in more pepper. Put some of the paste on your finger and rub it into the inside of the throat and all around the affected area. A lot of saliva will be produced. You can either swallow it or spit it out. This will help heal the inflammation and improve the health of your vocal cords.

Sesame Oil Bath for Arthritis & Rheumatism

Here is another simple health secret from a natural source. In India most people do this regularly, but the practice is almost unknown in the West. It is to apply sesame oil all over the body, leave it on for half an hour and then wash it off. The oil could be applied to the hair and scalp also. This provides a complete lubrication for the body, and will take care of many ailments. It helps to take away the toxins from arthritis and rheumatic troubles, and should be done at least once a week.

Natural Soaps

I would recommend that you avoid using soap as much as possible. Soap is made from caustic soda, which dries the skin. Even if oil is added to the soap, the caustic soda is still there. If you have very oily skin, you can wash with a paste of chickpea (garbanzo bean) flour. Just apply it to the body, let it dry and then rinse it off. Another cleansing paste can be made of fine mung bean powder and water. Even if your body is thoroughly soaked in oil, this paste will take it all away without harming the skin. If your skin is not oily, and you do the oil bath mentioned above, you do not even need to use soap; just shower and towel away the excess oil. The skin will remain moist. This is much more effective than using commercial creams.

CHAPTER 13:
FOOD & YOGA PRACTICE

For the full-time, serious student of Yoga, diet takes on another significance. The fifth limb of Raja Yoga is *pratyahara* or sense control. The tongue is the most powerful of the senses, and the most difficult to control. It has two functions: eating and talking. The Indian saint Ramalinga Swamigal advised that, "If a spiritual seeker is interested in food and eating, all of his spiritual practices will be like so many things thrown into a river. The benefits will all be washed away." Without control of the tongue you can forget about spirituality; you will not be able to control any of the other senses. All of the senses, even the sexual urge, can be controlled if you control your tongue.

How much time we waste constantly thinking of ice cream and pizza. In ashrams in India they serve the same food every day. The seekers there need not even bother to ask what the menu is each day. As long as it is good for the stomach, it will do. Saint Ramalinga said, "It does not matter what you feed me, Lord. When I am hungry, whatever comes to me, whatever is offered, let me just eat. I only want to serve You. I do not even want to look at what is offered. Whatever it is, I will simply put it in my mouth, chew it, swallow it, and be finished. I will say, 'Okay, body, I have paid you your due, now don't bother me anymore.'" This is the attitude of a true spiritual seeker. If one day there is nothing to eat, fine. "Well, God, probably that is Your will for me today."

The monks in India have some very simple rules about food. Right at noon each one is to take their begging bowl, go in front of a householder's house and stand there for the time it would take a capable person to milk a cow. (When these rules were thought of there were no clocks or watches.) They are to simply say once, "*Bhavati, bhiksham dehi*"—"Please give me some alms." If there is no response, they may go to another house, but with a limit of seven houses. If they get enough at the first house, they need not go farther.

But if they do not get anything even after seven houses, then they take it that the Goddess did not want them to eat that day. And that is not all. If they do get some food, they are to go to the riverbank, sit down and look here and there to see if anyone is around. If they see one or two people, they offer them as much as they want to eat. If there is anything left over, the monk may eat it. If five people come and eat it all, their attitude is: "I see, God came in five different forms and ate everything. I have been blessed, and God wants me to fast today."

I am not saying that you should take up a begging bowl tomorrow. But you should have that attitude, "Yes, God will give me whatever is necessary." If you are really serious about the yogic path, keep your food simple and just eat it and be done with it.

When you are fasting, keep the mind well occupied with things other than food. Do more Yoga practices; do not even give yourself time to think about food. That is real fasting. You are then also keeping your mind away from food. If you keep your body away from food but still fill the mind with it, you are not really fasting.

It is especially important to keep the stomach light if you want to meditate. Meditation means focusing the mind on one point with total concentration, and for this you need all your energy. When you eat, at least part of your energy immediately rushes to the stomach to digest the food. If you eat a lot, you will need all of your energy to go there. If you try to meditate, your energy gets confused: "What should I do now? Digest the food or help you meditate? Well, probably you can use your mind later but the food should not be left undigested so I'll go there first."

Then the brain becomes dull and you feel like sleeping instead of meditating. Again, this is why the tradition for so many religious holidays is to fast or eat lightly, so that you can spend your energy in prayer and meditation. If you want to be en-light-ened, keep the stomach light.

If your system is pure and strong, you will be able to digest anything. You will be immune to all the minor ailments and allergies. Your digestive fire will also be strong. Sometimes people tell me, "I have been following your suggestions and have made my diet very simple and pure. But instead of becoming stronger, I have become overly sensitive. If I go off my diet even a little, I immediately develop some physical symptoms or fall sick. What is happening to me?"

To this I must say, that is the problem with Yoga! If a glass of water is already dirty and you throw in more dirt, it will scarcely be noticeable. Or if you put on your dirty jeans and go do some greasy job, the new dirt will not show. But if you start with clean, pure water, even a speck of dirt will be visible; or if you wear all white clothes, even a tiny spot of grease will show.

If you smoke three packs of cigarettes a day and your lungs are filled with nicotine, smoking a cigarette, or even a whole pack, is nothing to you. But after you have practiced Yogic breathing for a few weeks or months and have eliminated the nicotine from your lungs, if you get even a small whiff of cigarette smoke, you will feel as if you are suffocating.

It is the same with yogic diet. A clean body will notice even a little heavy or unclean food and will be affected by it. But that is only until it becomes completely clean and strong. After a certain stage, you can even eat anything you want and not be affected. A young plant needs a fence around it until it grows into a tree. Once it is fully grown, not only does it not need the fence, but it can give shade to the other plants and to animals. Be gentle with your body until it really becomes strong. You may think, "I have been so good this whole week, now I deserve to celebrate a little and have some ice cream and cake;" but you should know that what is a celebration to you might well be a torture for your body.

It may inspire you to hear of a spiritual vow that many people take in India. I am not talking about the monks now, but about the simple village people. Lord Vishnu is said to use a golden eagle named Garuda for a vehicle. Therefore, whenever his devotees see a golden eagle, they are reminded of him. Many of them take a vow called "Seeing the Golden Eagle." This means they will not eat on that day until or unless they see a golden eagle. On some days they might not see one until three or four o'clock in the afternoon. Other days they might not see one at all; on those days they do not take any food. I have met people who have kept this vow for thirty or forty years. That is control over the tongue.

CHAPTER 14:

CONCLUDING THOUGHTS

We learn many things from the animals and birds. They eat simple, natural food and never have to go to the doctor. They never need pills for constipation or insomnia, or to get rid of gas. It is because they live according to nature. Mahatma Gandhi used to say very often, "Go back to nature. You will enjoy everything that is good in life." Our society has become unnatural in so many respects: our food is artificial, our dress is artificial, even so much of our thinking has become artificial. That is why we have so many problems—personal, interpersonal, national, international.

The aim of Yoga is to go back to nature as much as possible. To lead a natural life, with simple food, simple dress, simple living. Then naturally, the mind also will have high thinking. Once we start living simply, we will have the time to think high and to easily solve all our personal and world problems.

Let there be a limitation in everything, a tranquility in everything. As the *Bhagavad Gita* says, "Yoga is not for the person who eats too much, nor for the one who fasts excessively." Going to extremes can sometimes be easier, but the middle path is what we need for a life of health and peace. Let us think in a peaceful way; eat in a peaceful way. Let all of our actions be done in this spirit. Let us be easeful, peaceful, and useful.

PART III:

YOGIC DIET

By Reverend Kumari de Sachy, Ed.D.

and Carole Kalyani Baral, M.S.

CHAPTER 15:

YOGA PHILOSOPHY

Section 1 by Rev. Kumari de Sachy, Ed.D.

Swami Satchidananda called his approach to Yoga "Integral Yoga," that is, the Yoga of synthesis. Integral Yoga takes into consideration all aspects of the individual—the physical, emotional, mental, intellectual, social, and spiritual—exemplifying the branch of Yoga known as Raja Yoga. Although Raja Yoga (*raja* is Sanskrit for "royal") is generally thought of as the path of meditation that leads to control of the mind, effectively this branch of Yoga represents an integral approach to life.

Raja Yoga takes into account the entire life of the individual, its ultimate aim being the "total transformation of a seemingly limited physical, mental and emotional person into a fully illumined, thoroughly harmonized and perfected being—from an individual with likes and dislikes, pains and pleasures, successes and failures, to a sage of permanent peace, joy, and selfless dedication to the entire creation."

Yoga Sutras of Patanjali

The principal text of Raja Yoga is Patanjali's *Yoga Sutras*. The nearly 200 *sutra*s, or threads of meaning, are apportioned into four sections. The first, *Samadhi Pada*, or the Portion on Contemplation, presents the theory of Yoga and a description of the most advanced levels of the practice of *samadhi*, which is translated into English as "contemplation" or the "superconscious state." The second section, *Sadhana Pada*, the Portion on Practice, offers philosophy of a more practical nature. In this section, Patanjali expounds on the "eight limbs of Yoga." The third section, *Vibhuti Pada*, is the Portion on Accomplishments, and it describes the powers and accomplishments that can be achieved by the dedicated practitioner. The fourth and final section is called *Kaivalya Pada*, the Portion on Absoluteness, which discusses Yoga philosophically from the cosmic perspective.

The section most relevant to Swami Satchidananda's teachings on vegetarianism is the second one, the Portion on Practice. In this section, Patanjali lists the eight stages of Yoga practice. He refers to these stages as the "eight limbs," which is why the *Yoga Sutras* are also known as Ashtanga Yoga, or Eight-limbed Yoga. He lists these eight stages in the following order:

> *Yama* (abstention): non-violence, truthfulness, non-stealing, continence, and non-greed
>
> *Niyama* (observance): purity, contentment, accepting but not causing pain, study of spiritual books and worship of God or self-surrender
>
> *Asana* (posture)
>
> *Pranayama* (breath control)
>
> *Pratyahara* (sense withdrawal)
>
> *Dharana* (concentration)
>
> *Dhyana* (meditation)
>
> *Samadhi* (absorption or superconscious state)

The order of this listing is not arbitrary. Rather, it delineates an intentional, stage-by-stage approach that serves to guide Yoga practitioners in their pursuit of Self-realization. While each of the eight limbs is equal to the others and each is a necessary practice, notice that the first two limbs are *yama* and *niyama*. Why did Patanjali place them at the top of his list? Because *yama/niyama* form the moral and ethical foundation upon which all the other practices must rest, thus ensuring that any resulting accomplishments are used constructively for the good of the practitioner, and everyone else.

Yogic or Sattvic Food

To fully understand Swami Satchidananda's teachings on the relationship between Yoga and diet, specifically, the psychological and spiritual benefits of a vegetarian/vegan diet, it's important to know something about the three *gunas*, or the qualities of nature.

The philosophy behind the concept of the *gunas* is set forth in Book I, *sutra* 16, of Patanjali's *Yoga Sutras*: *Tat Param Purusa Khyater Gunavaitrsnyam*. In English: "When there is non-thirst for even the *gunas* (constituents of nature) due to realization of the *Purusha* (true Self), that is supreme non-attachment."

In his commentary on the *Yoga Sutras*, Swami Satchidananda wrote that, originally, the world, or *Prakriti* in Sanskrit, was *avyakta*, unmanifested. When *Prakriti* began to manifest, the ego came first; then, individuality emerged; and, finally, the mind materialized. From the mind, the *tanmatras* (a term that signifies the essence of objects) appeared, followed by the gross elements. This, from the yogic standpoint, is our natural evolution.

Yoga says that God is pure consciousness and *Prakriti*, the world, is there, too, its nature being to evolve and then to dissolve. *Prakriti*, in its unmanifested state, has both matter and force.

When nature is in an unmanifested condition, the force is static or dormant. This force, or *prana*, has three components called the *gunas*: *rajas*, *tamas*, and *sattva*, or the active state, the passive state, and the tranquil state, respectively. When all three of these qualities are in equilibrium, they don't affect matter. But even a little disturbance in the *gunas* creates motion in matter, giving rise to all the various forms; and that is how the entire universe, with all its elements, appears.

We can observe the *gunas* at work—and at play—in our personalities and even in the food that we eat. That is to say, some people are very active, even restless; others are slow and sluggish; and there are those who are tranquil and composed. In fact, in one of the principal scriptures of Yoga, the *Bhagavad Gita*, Lord Krishna offers a lengthy discourse on the various temperaments and the types of foods that attract them.

First, he describes calm people and their preferred diet:

> "Those of tranquil temperament [*sattvic*] prefer foods that increase vitality, longevity and strength; foods that enhance physical health and make the mind pure and cheerful; foods with substance and natural flavor; foods that are fresh, with natural oils and agreeable to the body." (17:8)

In his commentary on the *Bhagavad Gita*, Swami Satchidananda explains that Lord Krishna describes for us the nature of *sattvic* foods: they enhance vitality, vigor, energy, good health, and joyfulness; they are tasty and fresh, with a little oil (sesame and sunflower seeds, for example), and easy to digest.

Then, Krishna talks about restless people and their favorite foods:

> "Those of a restless, compulsive temperament [*rajasic*] prefer foods that are very spicy or very sour, piping hot, bitter, dry, or quite salty. Such foods give rise to discomfort, pain and disease and, therefore, dismay." (17:9)

Referring to Lord Krishna's comments about the deleterious effects of *rajasic* foods, Swami Satchidananda stressed that it isn't necessary to eat extremely spicy, hot food. He reminded us that just because Yoga comes from India, it doesn't mean that if we practice Yoga, we need to copy everything that's done in India. As a matter of fact, he said, eating hot food even once in awhile isn't that good for us, because as much as a day or two after eating very spicy food, we may feel our entire alimentary canal burning.

And from a more subtle perspective, Yoga teaches that if we're practicing meditation, it's better to refrain from eating spicy foods because these foods agitate the mind, making it difficult for us to meditate.

There has been a lot of discussion about the elimination of onions and garlic in a yogic diet. Swami Satchidananda was not opposed to them, in moderation, and not mainly added for purposes of taste. Rather, he often recommended their inclusion during the flu season. Onions and garlic do have some beneficial antiviral and antibiotic properties. They also can be helpful to control blood pressure and curb high cholesterol.

Swami Satchidananda often recommended *rasam*, a South Indian soup made with lentils, water, tomato, black pepper and other spices, and tamarind pulp. *Rasam* is very good for when one has a cold, as black pepper can help to control cold symptoms.

He also said that for stomach problems South Indian mothers added more turmeric to their dishes, because turmeric is a good antiseptic. To treat inflammations, they add something sour. We can use food, he said, as medicine; but medicine should be taken only as needed, not just because the tongue likes it.

Certain yogis believe onions and garlic are just too exciting to the senses—particularly for those who wish to practice celibacy—and therefore do not add value to their diets. Some substitute ginger, turmeric, and *asafetida* (or "hing" powder), which is a digestive aid with numerous medicinal properties; and, it adds a delicious flavor to foods.

Lastly, Krishna describes the lethargic types and their culinary preferences:

> Those of a dull and lazy temperament [*tamasic*] choose foods that are stale and tasteless, overcooked or left overnight, spoiled, rotting or even putrid. Such foods have lost their vitality and nutrition (17:10).

Generally, foods that are old, overcooked, very cold, or moldy fall into the *tamasic* category.

Concerning the relationship between food and the mind, while certain personality types are attracted to particular kinds of food, conversely, these same foods directly affect the personality. For example, in the *Bhagavad Gita*, Lord Krishna tells us that *rajasic* food creates restlessness in the mind. Thus, if our goal is to keep our mind calm and to remain peaceful, we wouldn't want to eat a lot of hot, spicy food or use too much garlic and onion. And, we wouldn't eat meat, which makes us active in a restless, sometimes aggressive manner.

Likewise, if we wish to remain alert and active, then we should stay away from those heavy, oily, overcooked, mind-numbing *tamasic* foods that make us dull and boring.

Swami Satchidananda taught that the manner in which we eat can also create a body and mind that is *sattvic, rajasic,* or *tamasic*. As an example, if we don't chew *sattvic* food well, it will ferment in the body and may result in *tamas*, or lethargy. Also, if we overeat right before going to sleep, we will become *tamasic*.

So, if you want to enjoy a balanced mind, a dynamic personality, a healthy body, and a peaceful and productive life, take the advice of the great yogis, past and present: make your diet a *sattvic* one. And always remember that diet shapes not only the body, but also the mind and the spirit.

Section 2 by Carole Kalyani Baral, M.S.

Prayerful Eating

In almost every culture there are different ways to say prayers before consuming food. Most of these prayers offer an opportunity to express the gratitude we feel to have the food we are about to eat. They sometimes give us pause to also reflect upon those who are less fortunate and may not be blessed with a bountiful abundance or variety of foods. Praying together reminds us that we are a family, a community, one world.

Before each meal at Satchidananda Ashram–Yogaville, and at all Integral Yoga Institutes and Centers, a meal prayer is recited. The prayer is in the ancient Sanskrit language, renowned for its profound and calming vibrational qualities. By offering a prayer before meals, we are reminded of several things: We eat to live (rather than living to eat). We have gratitude for the many blessings in our lives. We take a few moments to calm the mind and prepare the body to receive nourishment.

This meal prayer was composed in the 8th Century by the great sage Adi Shankaracharya. The prayer is then followed by the English translation, given by Sri Swami Satchidananda*:

Annapūrṇe Sadāpūrṇe
Śankara Prāna Vallabhe
Jñāna Vairāgya Sidhyartham
Bhiksham Dehī Cha Pārvati
Mātā Cha Pārvati Devī
Pitā Devo Maheśvaraha
Bāndhavāḥ Śiva Bhaktāha
Svadeśo Bhuvana Trayam

Hari OM Tat Sat Brahmāpaṇamastu
Lokāḥ Samastāḥ Sukhino Bhavantu
Jai Srī Sat Guru Mahārāj Ki! Jai!

OM Beloved Mother Nature,
You are here on our table as our food.
You are endlessly bountiful, benefactress of all.
Please grant us health and strength,
wisdom and dispassion,
to find permanent peace and joy,
and to share this peace and joy
with one and all.
Mother Nature is my mother.
My father is the Lord of all.
The whole creation is my family.
The entire universe is my home.
I offer this unto OM, that truth which is universal.
May the entire universe be filled with
peace and joy, love and light.
May the Light of Truth overcome all darkness.
Victory to that Light!

*Hear Sri Swami Satchidananda recite the meal prayer here: www.yogaville.org (search: meal prayer).

Sacred Food Offerings

In the Integral Yoga tradition, after a *puja* (worship service) food that has been offered first to the deities or saints is consumed afterward by the participants. Partaking in *prasad* (blessed food) is a gracious gift. For those who may like to include this in their

Yoga practice, several examples of fine vegetarian/vegan offerings for *prasad* might include:

Fresh organic fruit
Healthy cookies or crackers
Dried fruits and/or nuts
Stuffed fruit (such as dates with nut butter, pecan, and flaked coconut)
Other sweets (such as date-nut balls, see recipe section)

Another aspect of food offering is welcoming new residents to one's neighborhood—the iconic casserole is brought to the new home as a gesture of hospitality. A wonderful offering of food is when we prepare and bring food to the ill who are unable to feed themselves. Collections or foods for food banks and soup kitchens across the nation are a grand example of sharing the gifts we have been blessed to receive with others less fortunate than ourselves.

In the spirit of Yoga, those who cook for their families or others, ideally see themselves as selflessly serving and contributing to the health and well-being of those served. Therefore, a yogic attitude of peace and harmony would be established in the kitchen during the preparation of the food. A meditative attitude is what you will see in the kitchens of Satchidananda Ashram and Integral Yoga centers because it is understood that what goes into the meal is not just the ingredients but also the vibration in which it was created. A yogic cook will remember this during the process and carry the task with a loving heart and balanced mind.

CHAPTER 16:
YOGIC DIET GUIDELINES

While there may be many variations on the definition of a yogic diet, Swami Satchidananda taught that a yogic diet includes food sources that nourish the body and elevate the mind. This kind of food, infused with the element of *prana*—that which fosters vitality, strength, and clarity—is proper nourishment for us. The yogic philosophy also directs us to the concept of *sattva* (tranquility), which is created by following *ahimsa*, non-harming or non-violence. A yogic diet is a pure vegetarian or vegan diet and it includes so many varieties and genres of glorious edibles grown in harmony with nature's laws.

When we eat foods grown or prepared with an attitude of reverence for life, we increase our individual capacity for absorbing the *prana* to create a higher state of consciousness within us. We suggest organic or even veganic gardening as the method of choice for growing living foods. Below is a list of suggested foods that fit this qualification and are suitable for consumption by those on a yogic path. We will go into this more in depth in the next section (Part IV). Remember that the yogic approach is to view food as medicine to nourish and heal our bodies and calm our minds.

Recommended foods:

  Fruits and vegetables
  Whole grains
  Beans and legumes
  Tofu and soybean products
  Plant-based oils (sunflower, sesame, olive)
  Seeds and nuts (not salted or overly roasted)
  Maple syrup, agave, blackstrap molasses, stevia

Herbal teas
Sweet and savory spices
Sprouted seeds, beans or grains

Undesirable foods and substances:

Certain foods should be avoided because they have certain properties that can disturb the peace of our systems biologically or emotionally.

Foods from animal origins, including eggs
Animal fats (oils and spreads)
Fried foods
Highly processed or refined junk foods, sodas
White flour and sugar products
Canned foods (except tomatoes naturally preserved, and BPA free canned organic beans)
Stale or reheated foods that have been overly cooked
Foods cooked in microwaves
GMO originated grown foods
Alcohol, tobacco, stimulants, non-prescription or recreational drugs

White flour has been used for centuries, when mixed with water, as a type of glue. Imagine this product as it creates a coating in the digestive system preventing true absorption of good bacteria and nutrients. Much has been researched on the harmful effects of white sugar, which causes obesity, high glucose levels attributing to diabetes, and affects the liver adversely. Fried foods also wreak havoc by pouring harmful excess fats into one's delicate system. Genetically tampered foods can damage our ecosystems and eventually may show up in our genetic codes for generations to follow. Choose the ingredients for your meals wisely as there is so much at stake.

These yogic dietary principles are meant only as a guide for your own health needs. It is very easy to adopt a fanatical attitude in the name of Yoga and spirituality, especially in relation to one's diet. Swami Satchidananda cautioned against fanaticism and stressed moderation; rather than preaching vegetarianism and yogic diet to others, lead by example. He was a broad-minded person who knew that we all have to make our own choices according to several principals:

Individual constitutions and personal health
The season and climate in which we live
What foods are available locally
How the food is prepared and by whom
When food is eaten and where
How much is consumed for one's ability to digest

One of our biggest challenges in this area is actually our over-abundant variety of foods available in many countries. Over consumption of anything, no matter how well prepared, can be detrimental to one's health. Eating too much at one time or during one day can overload and cause damage to our bodies. Stagnation or slowing down of digestion creates dis-ease. Therefore moderation and judgment is employed to select, arrange, and provide proper nourishment to fulfill your role in this lifetime.

Have compassion for yourself when you veer off the path and, as quickly as possible, return to the principles of the yogic diet. Practicing *ahimsa* toward ourselves prevents harshness in our attitudes and welcomes a joyful outlook. It takes strength and fortitude to stay on a healthy path no matter how much knowledge we have. There is always room for learning and growth. The reward is a body and mind of optimal health, rooted in a spiritual approach to life.

Living a yogic lifestyle is an evolutionary journey during which we can strive to bring our bodies and minds into balance in all ways. In the next section, Dr. Sandra McLanahan will help guide us toward that balance.

PART IV:

GETTING STARTED:
HOW TO EAT WELL TO LIVE WELL

by Sandra Amrita McLanahan, M.D.

CHAPTER 17:

BALANCED DIET, BALANCED LIFE

Good health is not automatically guaranteed just because you are a vegetarian or a vegan. No doubt, going veg is a step in the right direction; but one of the most important and central principles for good health is moderation—in diet and in your attitude in life.

A balanced diet means not taking anything to the extreme. Even the best ingredients in a diet may not make you healthy if you don't eat in a conscious, moderate, and relaxed way.

What Not to Eat

Four major medical studies have now shown that if serum cholesterol is lowered by dietary changes, the incidence of heart disease goes down. It is possible to prevent heart attacks by following a changed diet. Regression and reversal can also be attained.

In populations that follow a plant-based diet, the heart attack rate remains low, even when there is severe stress, such as war. Our health does best if we eat a plant-based diet. If we put fats into our long intestinal tract, the body absorbs too much fat, and by the time we are eleven or twelve years old our arteries are streaked with fat. This process can begin as early as age two.

In addition, fats slow down the transit time of food through the bowels, again increasing the time these materials are in contact with the bowel wall, so that more fats are absorbed. Fats in the diet may also affect the balance of hormones in our bodies. A high-fat, low-fiber diet has been linked to appendicitis, diverticulitis, colitis, osteoporosis, cataracts, arthritis, heart disease, strokes, diabetes, and cancers of the breast, uterus, prostate, ovary, colon, and rectum.

Fats in the diet may call forth an increase in bile salts, digestive agents, which are known to be cancer-causing substances. Meat diets are much higher in saturated fat —a type of fat more resistant to processing by the body and therefore more likely to clog the arteries. Saturated fats also increase inflammation, a root cause of many chronic diseases. Cancer of the colon may be directly linked to the amount of saturated fat in the diet. Populations that eat such diets—especially diets high in beef—have a more elevated incidence of this cancer.

Plant sterols—complex hormone-like plant proteins—lower levels of cholesterol in the blood. Refined sugar, white flour, and white rice have now also been strongly linked to heart disease and cancer.

When to Eat

It would be ideal if our appetites could be our guides. Unfortunately, our often overly-sedentary lives do not allow us to take in all that we would like to without ill effects.

It is best to ingest most of the calories in the earlier part of the day. Research has concluded that calories consumed earlier in the day cause less weight gain than the same amount eaten later in the day. The process of digestion slows down significantly as the day progresses, and even more dramatically during sleep.

Sri Swami Satchidananda's recommendations for a daily meal plan that consists of a light breakfast, main meal for lunch and light dinner, make the most sense. After a period of seven hours or more of "fasting" during the night, it is a good idea to "break-fast," as Sri Swamiji says, with just a beverage or fruits. For some people who are doing heavy physical labor, this may not be advisable, but for those following a more sedentary life, it seems highly favorable. The noon meal is the best time for the largest caloric intake of the day, with plenty of time in the remaining day, to digest and burn off the calories. Supper should be early.

In one study, persons of normal weight were placed in a room with obese persons, and the clock on the wall was sped up. When the clock showed 12:00 noon—although in reality it was only 10:30 a.m., the overweight people generally took out their lunches and began to eat. Those who were at a more correct weight did not eat. We do best not to let the time of day rule our eating habits, but instead let our bodies and real appetite be our guide.

What to Eat

We've determined that a plant-based diet is optimal for human beings to digest and assimilate. But it is not enough to say that by abstaining from meat, fish, dairy, and eggs, one will be healthy.

The most simple and clear way to decide what is useful, from all the nutritional advice that abounds for vegetarians, vegans, or even non-vegetarians, is to use the principle: "Eat what is natural." This means to eat, as much as possible, foods as they occur in nature. "Organically Grown," "Whole Foods," "No Preservatives," "No Additives" are all labels that describe natural foods.

Foods can be prepared in a way that preserves their natural state as much as possible. Fruits are best taken raw. Vegetables can be taken raw or lightly steamed. If we eat an apple, our blood sugar stays at a nice and steady level within the normal range. If we eat applesauce, the blood sugar rises above the normal range, then falls. When the blood sugar is above normal, our white cells are less active to fight infection, inflammation, clots, or cancerous cells.

Pectin is higher in a vegetarian/vegan diet. Pectin is a complex carbohydrate found in many fruits. One study showed a 5 percent drop in cholesterol in just three weeks when 15 grams of pectin (the usual veg diet level) was given daily. Apples are high in pectin. An apple a day may very well keep the doctor away!

Whole foods are unprocessed foods. When rice is refined, the bran and germ are taken out and the majority of nutrients and fibers are lost. Whole grains are an essential part of the human diet and have been found to lower risk for heart disease and cancer. Removal of fiber from goods by processing—as is done with white flour or white rice—has been implicated in the development of appendicitis, diverticulosis and diverticulitis, colitis, hemorrhoids, varicose veins, gall stones, cancer of the colon, and diabetes. A vast amount of evidence now supports the thesis that whole foods prevent a wide variety of illnesses.

Dr. Denis Burkitt has called the United States "the most constipated country in the world." A high fiber, vegetarian diet can provide the daily bowel movement that avoids sludging in the bowel. That regularity is thought to reduce risk of colon cancer.

Fiber is that portion of the food that passes through the digestive tract without being absorbed. Fiber in the diet has many protective properties. It decreases the amount of carbohydrate that we absorb from our food and probably assists in protection from diabetes or allows diabetes to be treated more effectively once present. Fiber in the diet increases the amount of fat that passes through and out the digestive system, decreasing the amount of fat that is actually absorbed and thus may block the arteries. Increased fiber has been found to lower the level of low-density cholesterol—the "bad" cholesterol most associated with fatty buildup in the arteries.

Returning to a whole, natural, vegetarian or vegan diet can be a surprising delight. The result is an easefulness of the bowels and corresponding ease of other body functions.

How Much to Eat

Animal studies have shown doubled and tripled lifespans in groups fed a low-calorie diet. The diseases of aging and disturbed immunity were avoided: diabetes, cardiovascular deterioration, renal disease, cancer. Overweight human females have 8–10 times the rate of cancers of the uterus and breast. Over two-thirds of Americans are overweight. About one-third are enough above their ideal weight to cause serious disease such as high blood pressure, diabetes, and gall bladder diseases with attendant chronic disability and shortened life expectancy.

The excess consumption of fats and refined foods, may impair our immune status. In one study, persons fed a high protein meat-based diet had an increase in malaria, tuberculosis, and brucellosis.

On the other hand, fixation upon diet and weight can lead to so much stress in the mind, it may manifest as a disease itself. With consideration to constitutional factors, an ideal weight cannot merely be taken from a table, but is best formulated by a combination of risk factors, psychological and social aspects, and medical assessment, forming a holistic view.

One of the worst problems, of course, is knowing just how much to eat or even how to stop eating once we've begun. This is a matter of discipline and awareness that can be cultivated by practice. Techniques such as using a small plate or bowl and taking just the right amount of food, then washing the dish immediately after eating and moving onto a pleasant activity, may help keep the mind from temptations to overeat.

Becoming more in tune with our bodies and developing willpower so we are the masters instead of the slaves to our own desires are very desirable goals. Yoga practice can be especially helpful for those people who want to develop this kind of inner strength. What is particularly unique about Yoga is its ability to offer a good overall approach to preventive medicine. The basic program trains the body and mind to be under your control and helps you to be able to replace harmful habits with positive actions and attitudes. Once established in this lifestyle, you can automatically become a healthy vegetarian or vegan.

How to Eat

It is not just the type of food or the quantity of food, but the attitude and lack of stress with which we take our food that determines its ultimate effect.

To facilitate greater awareness of how and why we eat, it may be useful to keep a "Diet Awareness Chart." List the date, time, location, and mood you are in whenever you eat something. This will heighten your consciousness and may help you to have more control in determining when and how you will eat.

When you eat, it's an important practice in increasing your awareness and in aiding digestion, to slow down. "Chew liquids and liquify solids" is an ancient adage that is full of practical wisdom. It may help to make a determined effort to find a quiet spot where you can concentrate on eating and not engage in conversation. It has been shown by some ingenious laboratory experiments that the body works best if it can focus its blood supply at the digestive tract after food is put there.

Remember that the main function of eating is to preserve the strength of the physical form in order for us to maintain a healthy lifestyle.

CHAPTER 18:

THE MEDICAL BENEFITS OF FASTING

The unending, sometimes strange, stream of food materials thrust on the digestive system to sort out and assimilate, is often consumed without much reflection upon its effect on the magnificent instrument that is the human body.

Fasting is a way to assist the body in its maintenance and repair work. It can help rejuvenate your body and mind. Whenever you eat, a significant shift in blood supply goes down into the digestive tract, to attend to processes of digestion. Relatively less is given to the brain, making you feel sleepy after a meal. For this reason, many spiritual traditions recommend fasting as a means of staying more mindful and awake during religious holy days.

The old adage, "Starve a fever, feed a cold" is a result of a distortion by history. The original proverb was: "If you feed a cold, then you'll have to starve a fever." So the original message back then was, it is best to fast for both conditions. Time played the game "Telephone" with this useful proverb, making it into an urban myth.

Fasting for both makes physiological sense, since bacteria and viruses are more vulnerable to food deprivation than the body's cells. In addition, if the body does not have to send blood to digestion, it can focus its resources on fighting the infection. It's as if, when you stop taking guests in the front door (the mouth), your body is able to send resources to clean its closets (the tissue) to do whatever repair work your body needs to achieve.

Scientific studies have shown that fasting lowers the levels of circulating insulin, thus helping to prevent and treat metabolic syndrome and Type 2 diabetes. Fasting also lowers levels of Insulin-like Growth Factor (IGF-1); high levels are associated with increased rates of aging and cancer. Animals that engage in some fasting regularly live longer, and with less chronic disease.

Fasting has also been shown to increase levels of Brain Derived Neurotrophic Factor (BDNF); low levels are found in Alzheimer's disease. This factor acts like an antidepressant. In addition, fasting has been documented to lower blood pressure and elevate mood. In one study, fasting even one day per month lowered risk for a heart attack by 42 percent.

Perhaps if we always ate just the right foods, in just the right amounts, and with the right attitude, there would be less need to fast for health and healing. Then we could consider fasting only as a spiritual practice—for its ability to help with focusing the mind.

Fasting Guidelines

The liver stores enough protein for two weeks; do not fast for more than that, or your body will start to break down your own muscles to get protein.

1. Do not fast for more than a few days unless you check with your doctor.

2. Never fast without drinking plenty of water. You can also drink hot water with lemon and cayenne, ginger tea, or garlicky tomato soup.

3. Do not drink bottled fruit juices, though diluted fresh orange, grapefruit, or lemon juices are acceptable.

4. If you fast for more than one day, take an enema (plain water is fine) or liquid fiber such as Benefiber.

5. Fast one day a week; two-three days once a month; five to seven days once or twice a year.

6. Stop if you feel light-headed, or experience excessive fatigue.

7. Monitor your tongue, saliva, and appetite to determine how long to fast.

8. Take as many days as you fast to return to normal eating: start with fresh fruits, then vegetables, and finally grains and beans.

Fasting Recipes

1. Diluted fresh-squeezed fruit juices:
   Oranges, grapefruits, lemons, grapes, berries, apples
   (can add ginger, wheatgrass, spirulina)

2. Fresh-squeezed vegetable juices:
   Any vegetable, especially beets, cucumbers, carrots
   (can add ginger, wheatgrass, spirulina)

3. Zucchini-green beans mixture:
   (especially good for hypoglycemia)
   Chop zucchini and green beans, boil in plenty of water for five minutes, whiz in blender. Drink hot or cold all day long.

4 Dried greens:
   Green magma, Kyo-Green, Flora Udo's Choice Green Blend, Flora Udo's Choice Wholesome Fast Food

5. Fruit fast:
   Just watermelon, or other fruits
   (with occasional rice cake or air popped popcorn)

PART V:

MAKING THE TRANSITION

*by Carole Kalyani Baral, M.S. and
Rev. Prem Anjali, Ph.D.*

CHAPTER 19:
AN INTRODUCTION
TO HEALTHY CHOICES

If you are new to this diet, we would like to offer some basic and informative guidelines and instructions to assist you in your transition to a vegetarian/vegan whole foods diet.

Choosing organic foods is essential if you want to cut down your intake of the types of additives and toxins currently found in our soil. There's a new generation of small scale veganic farmers who try to avoid using all animal fertilizers and by-products in order to bring forth the best crops. These independent "renaissance" farmers are increasing and making it possible for us to eat the healthiest and purest products available to us at this time. Try to locate and support them in your community.

Later in this book, you will find suggestions for various vegetarian meals and recipes. Feel free to adapt and adjust these to suit your family and their needs. Many of our food choices and preferences seem to arise from what we have been used to eating throughout our lives. For this reason, it's so important for parents to introduce their children to new tastes and new types of food at an early age, so that later on they will be able to make their own healthy choices.

Part of transitioning to a healthier diet is trying new products and experimenting with different tastes and textures, making the changes part of an adventure. For example, the elimination of dairy products and eggs has become much easier than in previous decades because of the products that have been developed since the 1960s. The choices today are abundant and offer a tremendous variety of possibilities for the thoughtful diner. And, there are always new products on the horizon as the popularity of vegetarian and vegan foods keeps increasing, and as people become aware of the benefits of eating in a conscious, compassionate manner.

For those new to plant-based diets (and even for those who have been following this lifestyle for some time), you may wonder where to derive important nutrients like calcium, Omega 3s, as well as sources of protein, iron, and vitamins like B and C. The following list will help guide your choices so you can ensure that you are eating a well-balanced, nutrient-rich diet.

CHAPTER 20:

A WHOLESOME GUIDE TO GOOD NUTRITION

Building Strong Bones

Adzuki beans
Almond butter
Blackberries
Blackstrap Molasses
Broccoli
Dates
Dried apricots
Figs
Kale and other leafy greens
Oranges
Sesame seeds and tahini
Soy products (soymilk and tofu)
Sweet potatoes

Fish-free Omega 3s

Berries
Cauliflower
Chia seeds
Flax seeds
Hemp seeds
Herbs and spices (cloves, oregano, star anise, and tarragon)
Leafy greens
Mangoes
Seaweed (chlorella, nori, spirulina)
Walnuts

Healthy & Happy Vitamin C

Bell peppers
Broccoli
Brussels sprouts
Cauliflower
Citrus fruits
Herbs (some, such as basil, chives, cilantro, parsley, and thyme)
Kiwi fruit
Leafy greens
Strawberries
Tomatoes

Protein Powerhouses

Beans (black beans, chickpeas, kidney beans, etc.)
Buckwheat
Chia seeds
Green peas
Hemp products (hemp milk and hemp seeds)
Lentils
Nuts and seeds (almonds, cashews, pecans, pumpkin seeds, nut butters, sunflower seeds, tahini, walnuts, etc.)
Oats
Quinoa
Soy products (soymilk, soy yogurt, etc.)
Tempeh

Pumping Iron and Catching B's

Chlorella
Fortified foods (cereal, plant milks that aren't homemade, vegan yogurts)

Leafy greens
Marmite and other yeast extracts
Nutritional yeast
Nuts and seeds
Tofu
Tomato paste
Whole grains (brown rice, buckwheat, bulgur, quinoa,
            oatmeal, wheat, etc.)

CHAPTER 21:

BASIC INGREDIENTS

Flours

Whole wheat flour, made from the entire wheat berry, retains much of its important nutritional value when made into bread. Look for the label "stone-ground," which refers to the fact that the berries are ground by large grinding stones rather than by electric roller mills. The reason stone-ground flours are generally more expensive is that the grinding process takes longer to prepare for market.

Whole wheat pastry flour is made from soft wheat berries and is used for more delicate baking needs, especially in dessert recipes. Soy flour is also high in protein and is gluten-free. Wheat germ (use "raw") and bran (high in B complex vitamins) can always be added to whole wheat bread products to further boost their high fiber content; they also add trace minerals.

Gluten-free Products

Gluten is the substance present in cereal grains that is responsible for the elastic texture of dough and that traditionally holds bread together. Gluten is also the property that makes it possible to mold grains into a specific shape. Gluten, the mixture of two proteins, causes illness in those who have celiac disease because it triggers inflammation and possibly long-term damage in the small intestines. Therefore, those who suffer from celiac disease should carefully avoid eating products that contain gluten.

Many foods are naturally gluten-free: fruits and vegetables, beans and seeds, legumes and nuts. The grains that are gluten-free are:

amaranth, buckwheat, corn, rice (all forms), millet, quinoa, soy and teff. Oats are questionable because of their possible contamination at the factory or while being transported and should be avoided unless specifically labeled as certified gluten-free. Bean flours and pea flours are the newest addition to gluten-free eating and appear today in many protein powder drinks. In fact, look to the future of pea protein to be used as an inexpensive way to add high protein to many forms of vegetarian foods.

Today, there are many gluten-free prepared food options that can be especially helpful for those with celiac disease or gluten sensitivities. However, a small note here of caution is warranted when shopping for these products: Take care to read the list of ingredients as many of these products contain concentrated sweeteners and refined flours, so moderation is recommended.

Legumes and Beans

These foods are an ideal part of a healthy diet because they are low in fat, have no cholesterol, and are high in folate, which all vegetarians/vegans need. The *difference between* a *legume* and a *bean* is that a *legume* is a class of vegetables that includes *beans*. Try saying this fast three times: Although beans are always legumes, legumes aren't always beans! A legume is simply a plant with a fruit that grows in the form of a pod. Examples are peas, beans, and peanuts. A bean is just a seed of a certain variety of plant species. Some classic beans include green beans, lima beans, soybeans, chickpeas, adzuki, kidney, pinto, and black beans. This food source offers vegetarians and vegans a tremendous variety from which to choose.

There are two main ways to prepare beans. One is to sort them carefully, soak them overnight (discarding the soaking water to eliminate its gas-producing qualities), and then cook them for at least an hour in fresh water. This method is simple, inexpensive, and healthy, but, it takes effort. Make sure not to add salt to the cooking water or the beans will not get soft.

The second, and more convenient method is simply to buy canned beans. Look for "organic" and "BPA-free" on the label and brands that are preferably labeled "low salt." Also, by rinsing the canned beans you can reduce the salt content of any brand that has included salt in the cooking process.

Some legumes are erroneously called nuts. The most common are peanuts and soy nuts. These are high in protein but also contain a fair amount of fat. Choose dry-roasted, unsalted brands that avoid adding oil and salt which is not conducive to health. Look for those peanut and soy "butters" that are pure with no added sugars or other additives for maximum health and taste.

A more recently discovered vegan delight is called "aquafaba," a term that refers to the liquid accompanying canned chickpeas and other legumes. It can be used in a variety of ways to mimic egg whites in order to bind, gelatinize, and thicken ingredients in recipes and create a type of vegan meringue.

Lentils

These are popular in many Eastern countries, especially India (in the form of *dals*), as they are very high in protein, easily digestible for most people, and come in a variety of colors. Their flat round shape is different from that of most other legumes and they do not have to be soaked before cooking. Some varieties of lentils come in red, brown, yellow, and green and the nutritional value is high in all forms. Each type lends itself to different dishes depending on regional preferences. Many vegetarians/vegans depend on lentils to satisfy their protein intake, as lentils are inexpensive and easy to obtain in markets worldwide.

Nuts

There are so many varieties of nuts to enhance and excite the taste buds. Nuts contain natural oils and fats, deliciously presented in high nutrient value and exotic taste. Using pecans or walnuts in baking goods helps to augment the protein power of the dessert and adds flavor and texture to the product. Raw cashews have been discovered to make a fine nut milk and can be pureed for sauces and to thicken soups.

Although the raw form of the nut is usually better for health, the varieties of nuts that are roasted are tasty for garnishes and snacks. Pine nuts are delicious in salads and in pesto. Almonds are excellent when mixed with green beans and when added to vegetarian paté recipes.

For cooking purposes, soak the raw nuts in water first for at least 1 to 2 hours. Discard the water and then rinse the nuts well. Soaking renders the nuts more digestible and allows the enzymes to be neutralized so that the body can fully utilize their benefit.

Oils

Oils are necessary in order to add good fats to the diet. They help build healthy membranes and assist the intestines in absorbing vitamins. They keep the skin soft and aid in the elimination process. The best oils are the unsaturated choices, which have the necessary essential fatty acids such as Omega 3 and 6, that a healthy body craves.

For cooking: sunflower, safflower, soybean, olive, and sesame oils are preferred. First pressed imported olive oil adds a fine flavor to salads and raw vegetables. California is one of the major producers of fine oils because of the abundant sunlight and fields dedicated to these crops. Oils help lower cholesterol and are necessary for good brain function. Yet, oils should be used sparingly as they are contributors to high blood pressure and heart disease if used in excess. Organic spray oil from a can, is a convenient option and can help reduce the amount of oil used for cooking and coating pans. Spectrum brand is known for its high quality and careful processing methods.

Pastas

Pastas and noodles are very popular. They are convenient, enjoyable, and can be healthy comfort foods. Many ingredients have been added today to boost the nutritional value of these highly digestible foods. Look for whole grain pastas that are darker in color and have more accessible protein than the white variety. The Bionaturae brand creates whole grain pastas that are excellent in taste and texture. "Explore Asian" brand puts *edamame* (young soybeans) into their pasta, making it incredibly abundant in protein and flavor.

There are many newly designed bean pastas, like black bean and adzuki bean, that are truly satisfying when served with sauces or added to soups. The question, "Where can I get my protein?", can be easily answered with some pastas containing 24 grams of protein per serving!

There is also a whole plethora of Asian ramen, *soba*, and *udon* noodles that are prepared with buckwheat or yam flours. Rice noodles are gluten-free as are kelp (from seaweed) and cellophane (clear) varieties. These are easy to prepare either from the dried or fresh varieties, and they usually please the whole family. For every meal, each variety can be enhanced by creating different, tantalizing sauces to complement. The sophistication of noodle culture today makes noodles an absolutely wonderful addition to any vegetarian menu.

Peas

A number of legumes are labeled as peas, including green peas, snow peas, snap peas, split peas, and black-eyed-peas. They are high in protein and low in fat. Most peas have a naturally sweet flavor and are great as a side dish, as a snack, in stir-fry dishes and in salads.

Seasonings

There are many types of salts that add flavor and make foods so tasty. Sea salt, rather than regular table salt, is preferred as it is less refined because it's processed without the chemicals found in ordinary salt. Many salts, like Himalayan pink salt, are found in crystal form and added to food with the help of a salt grinder or a mill. Black salt has a distinctive taste—due to its sulfur content—that can mimic the taste of eggs in the vegan diet.

Since too much salt can be a health hazard, care should be taken to use this ingredient sparingly. The rule of thumb when it comes to salt: Taste first and then add if necessary.

Vegetable salts or salt substitutes are great for those who want to avoid salt for various reasons. Spike Vegit and Herbamare (look for the ones labeled "no salt") are two brands that are good tasting and contain similar salty flavors but from vegetables, seaweed, and spices. Sea kelp, used in a refined shaker form, can also be delicious. Kelp contains natural iodine, though this it is not to be considered "low sodium" for those on sodium-restricted diets.

Spices such as the following are flavorful and versatile helpers that turn everyday meals into special taste treats:

Turmeric powder flavors and adds a yellow color to tofu salad and has valuable anti-inflammatory properties; *garam masala* is a combination of many aromatic spices—cloves, cinnamon, nutmeg, cardamom, and black pepper—to flavor Indian dishes; saffron is the most pricey and exotic of seasonings and it's used to flavor and add color to rice dishes like Spanish-style *paella* and Indian delicacies. Additionally, you can explore the use of garlic and ginger to flavor foods.

There are many different forms of pepper as in cayenne, red, black, and white pepper that can add flavor and depth to many dishes. Brands like Frontier Food Co-op and The Spice Hunter, among others, have created incredible spice blends: Tagine (a Moroccan blend of spices), Fajita seasoning, Thai, African curry, Cajun seasonings, many Indian curry blends, and more. Check out Frontier's herbal blends too—Herbes De Provence, Herbs of Italy—as many of these blends are salt-free! You may be surprised to find stores in your area that you can explore that specialize in fresh and exotic herbs and spices.

Sea Vegetables

These gifts from the sea are wonderful and versatile and deliver trace minerals not found in land vegetables. However, for those on salt-restricted diets, a caution is in order because most are quite high in sodium.

The fiber and vitamins that sea vegetables contain—for instance, natural iodine—are crucial to our health and lacking in many of our diets.

Snacking on seaweed has become convenient; you can purchase packages of seaweed—mostly made from *nori*—in bite size sheets at health food stores or Asian markets. These packets make great food-on-the-go snacks and for children's lunchboxes.

Seaweeds can be crushed by hand to sprinkle on salads and soups to heighten any product that you consume, and they need no rehydration. Seaweeds are a real gift for your body and help the brain function properly. The varieties of seaweeds are endlessly abundant and add natural salt to your diet. Salt is necessary for your system to function properly, but, of course, those whose health issues require them to be on a salt-restricted diet, need to monitor their salt intake.

Nori: a toasted sheet of seaweed used for veggie rolls that are called sushi. *Nori* has a mild flavor and melts in your mouth. It can also be found in snack size packets for convenience.

Arame: a good tasting variety that comes in thin shredded strips. It is sweeter and milder than its cousin, *hiziki*, and when it's combined with carrots, onions, and celery, and served with brown rice, it makes a delicious dish.

Hiziki: a good choice to add to vegetables, salads, and soups. Highly nutritious, it contains abundant trace minerals plus iron and magnesium. It helps to control anemia as it raises the iron in blood.

Dulse: in it's flaked form, it can be sprinkled on salads. It is versatile as a powder and can be added to grain and vegetable dishes to increase the protein content. *Dulse* has a rather strong seaweed flavor.

Kelp: a good salt substitute when used in a fine powder form. There are 30 varieties that grow in kelp forests under the sea. It is high in calcium but also in sodium. Use kelp in moderation if you are watching your salt intake.

Kombu: found in long, broad strips, *kombu* can be used in soups and to cook beans. It can be used to help soften beans; and, because of its sea origin, it adds a salt-like flavor and trace minerals. Add *kombu* to make *miso* soup even more delicious by cutting it into thin strips after reconstituting it with cooking. You can create "the liquid of the gods" (called *dashi*) using *kombu*. This highly treasured broth is used abundantly in Japanese cooking.

Wakame: a form of seaweed that has a mildly sweet flavor and can be used in salads and miso soups. *Wakame* is a healthy favorite in Japanese cuisine in the form of seaweed salad, which usually contains rice vinegar and tamari sauce, plus ginger and perhaps sesame oil.

Seeds

Another valuable addition to our plant-based diet are seeds. Sunflower and pumpkin seeds are perfect in salads and on hot breakfast cereals. Hemp seeds are the new super food as they boost the protein of everything that they are added to, including shakes, baked goods, and granola. Chia and flax seeds can be soaked and used as egg substitutes for baking as they create a gelatinous binding agent.

Flax and sesame seeds can be used to make crackers or they can be ground to add phytonutrients to any cereal. Sesame seeds can be made into a paste called tahini, and tahini is often used to create delicious dressings included in Middle Eastern dishes. Sesame seeds are abundant in calcium and augment the nutritional value of dips and spreads—although these seeds are high in calories.

All seeds are packed with fiber, protein, good fats, and antioxidants. They help in weight reduction when added to a dish, as they make you feel fuller and more satisfied.

Soy Products

Since the soybean contains all nine essential amino acids that are necessary for health—and that cannot be manufactured by the body—it has been called the perfect food. In many parts of the world, populations that consume the amazing soybean rather than animal foods are thriving. In fact, soybeans were served to the survivors of nuclear explosions to help heal their lungs after exposure to the contaminants released by those explosions.

The variety of products made from the soybean includes tofu and tempeh, now found in abundant flavors and textures in every supermarket across the world. Miso is a fermented soybean paste that is used for flavorings and for healthy soups. It also comes in a large array of flavors and in assorted colors, making each product unique. Tamari is a naturally fermented soy sauce, which usually has no additives. It can be found in gluten-free and reduced sodium forms—even in sodium-reduced form, all tamari is high in sodium and should be used sparingly.

Other forms of the soybean are used to make products that resemble meat both in flavor and texture. Almost every product in the deli case of your local supermarket can be found in an analogous form—utilizing soy—in which no animal has been harmed. Soymilks are deliciously nutritious, as are *edamame* (Japanese-style young soybeans, which are good for snacks) and T.V.P. (textured vegetable protein), used for crumbles and burgers.

Sprouts

Sprouts may be considered the best form of raw food nutrition. By converting the seeds and beans that sprouts are made from into energy, enzymes are activated that aid digestion and create greater nutritional value. Sprouts contain iron, calcium, protein, and Vitamins B and C. It's as if the seed wakes up and starts to grow, with the water and the sun, into a viable food source high on the list for optimal survival.

There are numerous books and websites that can teach you to grow all types of sprouts, including, alfalfa, radish, green lentils, chickpeas, mung beans, sweet pea, and soybeans. Even cereals and vegetables can be sprouted to add to sandwiches, salads, and vegetable dishes. Keep sprouts refrigerated after sprouting and they should last for about a week. It's great to grow sprouts on your own, but you can also conveniently purchase them in a store, provided you check the dates carefully for freshness.

Also there are several Essene-type breads that are made from sprouts and are naturally sweet and contain no flour. These breads come in a variety of flavors with added dried fruits and /or nuts; they are easily digested and they are gluten free.

New cousins of sprouts that are now found in markets are microgreens, which are grown in soil and harvested without the roots. Microgreens add color, intricate designs, and particularly stronger flavors than sprouts. They take longer to grow (10 to14 days), but they are abundantly high in all nutrients. They are also used as garnishes for gourmet dishes. Imagine tiny greens grown from arugula, basil, beets, and kale gracing your table and coming from the most densely nutritious vegetables.

Sweeteners

We recommend using natural fruits—especially bananas, applesauce, berries, and dried fruits—to sweeten foods and baked goods. Sugar is available in so many cheap forms, but it harms the teeth by causing decay, and, it also increases body weight, because it stimulates insulin production contributing to diabetes. Additionally, sugar is called the food with "empty calories," as it contains no nutritional value. If one is to use sugar, turbinado (a darker sugar that is less processed and, therefore, healthier than regular white sugar) is preferable but should be used sparingly.

The most harmful form of sweetener is the high fructose corn syrup obtained from farmer's surplus and offered as a cheap additive to many foods. Beware of products that use this sweet filler, as it may be detrimental to your health. It is especially abundant as an ingredient in high calorie soft drinks. Thankfully, these soft drinks have been banned in many schools that once served them owing to studies that showed the negative impact these products had on students' health.

An abundant variety of naturally sweet products are available today. Wholesome options include: maple syrup (from trees), agave (from cactus plants), molasses (usually blackstrap from sugar process), and sorghum (from grain). Maple sugar can also be found in a granulated form, which is pricey but deliciously delicate in flavor and is used more as a sprinkled topping than as a baking ingredient.

Currently, stevia is the new sensation on the market. Stevia, which comes from the leaves of the plant, provides a very sweet product that contains no calories and does not raise one's glucose level. In the liquid form, Sweet Leaf brand is both versatile and delicious in beverages and on foods. It is available in many flavors (vanilla crème, root beer, clear, lemon, peppermint, grape, English toffee— to name a few) and adds natural goodness to whatever it graces.

The yogic principal of *ahimsa* (nonviolence) reminds us not to harm any living creature on this green earth. Sadly, however, for decades, we have been behaving inhumanely toward our honeybees, sacrificing them in order to provide us with products that we covet. For those who wish to follow a vegan diet, thankfully, there are so many sweeteners other than honey that are readily available.

Whole Grains

Whole grains are an important component of a healthy and wholesome diet, as they contain the entire bran, germ, and endosperm of a plant. In this form, whole grains retain a high protein factor as well as vast nutritional properties. They are the whole seed of the grain as it is grown in nature. Flours made from these grains are all high in fiber and other vitamins and minerals that encourage good health.

Some of the more popular whole grains are amaranth, barley, brown rice and wild rice, buckwheat, bulgur (cracked wheat), corn (including popcorn, a whole grain snack), millet, oats (including oatmeal), quinoa (varieties include white, red, and black grains), spelt, and teff (a grain used in Ethiopian cuisine).

Basmati brown rice emits a wonderful fragrance while being cooked and tastes delicious with Indian style vegetables and soups. Breads, pastas, and crackers made from these ingredients (and labeled as "whole") add substantial value to the diet when eaten in moderation, since they also contain high carbohydrate values.

Couscous, from wheat, is not a whole grain product and proves to have less nutritional content; however, couscous has some redeeming value for busy households, as it requires a minimum amount of preparation.

Combine:

| 1 cup | couscous |
| 1 cup | boiling water |

1. Cover for 10 minutes.
2. Use a little more water for a softer and stickier grain.
   Fluff with a fork and it is ready!

Couscous can be used to accompany vegetables and bean dishes since it absorbs sauces and gravies well. Israeli couscous, a whole grain, comes in a pearl form and resembles barley, is chewy in texture and has a nutty flavor. This form requires only about 10 minutes of cooking time and is deliciously different from other grains.

CHAPTER 22:

EASY-TO-USE SUBSTITUTES FOR ANIMAL-BASED FOODS

A new industry has been created for the millions of vegetarians/ vegans who are now choosing to eat a conscious diet of plant-based foods. Many of these products are convenience foods that have noteworthy nutritional value consisting of plant protein; they are easy to transform into full, delicious meals that are perfect for today's working families.

However, as with all convenience foods, check out the sodium content if you are on a salt restricted diet, as some are quite high in this ingredient. As you become more acclimated to a vegetarian diet, hopefully you will enjoy exploring the abundant varieties of ingredients, recipes, and resources, affording you the ability to choose the healthiest and most convenient food preparation opportunities.

We highly recommend a trip to your local natural/health food store, food co-op, or grocer. It will be fun and also greatly informative. Usually, the store manager or staff members can answer your questions or point you in the right direction so you can get the products that you need. Most non-perishables are also easily available online, and it's useful to note that many of the home delivery subscription services (Blue Apron, HelloFresh, Home Chef, Plated) offer vegetarian and even vegan options.

The following brands and their products are by no means an exhaustive listing or an endorsement—although we've tried them all and have tried to include what are, in our view, some of the best offerings. We hope this list provides you with some ideas and suggestions regarding tasty, convenient alternatives that will please the palate while allowing you to observe ethical principles.

Bacon

Lightlife's Smart Bacon is one of the best. Traditional (made from a pig!) bacon is hard to replicate in the veg world, but remember that it takes time to develop a taste for alternatives and that taking the time is worth it for your health, your heart, and your planet! Whether served up with scrambled eggs or topping off a veggie burger, Smart Bacon brings a hearty bacon taste to your meal, yet it's free of saturated fat and cholesterol. Yves Veggie Cuisine also makes a Canadian veg bacon.

Beef & Chicken

Brands like WestSoy have created various flavor seitans like "Chicken Style" and ground beef-like textures, as well as strips and cubes, which make great meat and poultry substitutes. Seitan is incredibly rich in vegetable protein and contains even higher values than tofu or tempeh. You can also buy the powdered mix and make your own seitan and freeze some for later use. Arrowhead Mills Vital Wheat Gluten is a good product to use to make this delicious delicacy.

Beyond Meat is a newer company that is been making a big splash with frozen foods like chicken strips and beef crumble from non-GMO soy and pea protein.

Gardein Products is a Canadian company that has totally revolutionized some old time favorites. They have an extensive array of excellent, no cholesterol, partially prepared frozen dishes, including Chick'n Scallopini. They all require a minimum amount of cooking and preparation and suit many customers' tastes.

Burgers & Hot Dogs

There is an abundant variety of prepared, frozen veggie burgers on the market today. If you're in the mood for something small and hearty in a hurry, Gardein's Ultimate Beefless Sliders give you the best of both worlds—they're packed with heart-healthy vegan protein and are made with simple natural ingredients, and they're ready in just a few minutes! They're also low in fat and made with non-GMO ingredients.

The newest kid on the block is Beyond Meat. This company makes the Beyond Burger and Beast Burger, a new breed of burgers made from pea protein and usually found in the meat aisle—because they've been called a "game changer" in terms of how close to a non-veg burger they are!

Boca Burgers and Gardenburgers have long been favorites among the veg community, as have been Amy's and MorningStar brands. Lightlife makes tempeh burgers and "Smart Patties" with quinoa or black beans. Some brands are lower sodium than others.

Lightlife created the original vegetarian hot dog, "Tofu Pups," and later added "Smart Dogs" to their line. Yves Veggie Cuisine soon followed with their line of "Tofu Dogs" and "Veggie Dogs." Great options for kids, too, because these dogs are quick and easy to prepare and perfectly paired with a whole grain hot dog bun, garnished with all the condiments.

Butter & Mayo

Earth Balance Organic Buttery Spread is the original vegan alternative to butter. This company has now expanded its line to include such spreads as soy-free, organic whipped, olive oil-based, and Omega-3. With the growing popularity of coconut oil, the most recent addition to the line is a coconut spread.

Miyoko's Kitchen, known for its gourmet approach to vegan foods (see "Cheeses"), has created a "Vegan Butter," a European style cultured butter that melts, cooks, bakes, and spreads like butter!

Just as Earth Balance is the gold standard in butter alternatives, Follow Your Heart's "Vegenaise" is the gold standard in vegan mayonnaise. Their latest offering is Sriracha Vegenaise! Since then, Hellmann's, the well-known mayo company, added their own vegan mayo to their line, as has Hampton Creek with their "Just Mayo." Nuco, a company with a line of coconut products, has a coconut vegan mayo.

Cake, Cookie, Pancake & Waffle Mixes

If you're looking for easy to prep mixes that don't call for eggs and are gluten-free, dairy-free, wheat-free, and nut-free, then Cherrybrook Kitchen is the answer! This company offers a line of mixes that include: Chocolate Chip cookies, Fudge Brownies, Yellow cake, pancakes, waffles, and frostings.

Cheeses

The vegan cheese industry has really grown over the last five years, creating delicious cheeses from almonds, cashews, and soy.

Creamy Cheeses and Dressings

The Daiya brand has a line of vegan cream cheeses and creamy dressings like Blue Cheeze, among others. Follow Your Heart offers vegan cream cheese and sour cream. Kite Hill has a vegan Brie made from almonds, which captures the tang and the consistency of the famous French cheese. They also offer a ricotta as does the Tofutti brand.

Meltable

The gold standard in "meltable" cheese (long the challenge for vegan cheeses) is the Daiya brand. Their mozzarella or cheddar shreds actually melt like dairy cheese and are perfect for pizza and nachos.

Field Roast Grain Meat Co.'s Vegan Chao Slices is a rich and creamy vegan cheese product that is coconut-based, seasoned with a fermented tofu, and traditionally called "Chao" by the Vietnamese. Chao Slices come in a variety of bold flavors, offering a cheesy bite right out of the package or melted on your favorite vegan sandwich or burger.

Slices, Cubes

Daiya offers vegan deli slices of such favorite cheese styles as cheddar, Swiss, or provolone. Daiya also has a line of vegan cheese cubes. Follow Your Heart also has an excellent line that includes smoked gouda and parmesan.

Nut cheeses

Miyoko's Kitchen has created gourmet, artisan cultured vegan nut cheeses—such as double cream sundried tomato garlic—with various flavors and textures. The creator received the 2016 "Vegetarian Hall of Fame" award given by North American Vegetarian Society.

Pizza Cheeses and Prepared Foods

There are numerous companies making frozen vegan pizzas with a variety of crusts and toppings. Daiya brand and Amy's are the leaders. Among other companies are Tofurky, BOLD Organics, and Ians. For those who prefer to dine out on pizza, many restaurants will often agree to allow you to bring in your own *unopened* (as per Health Department regulations) package of Daiya or other vegan alternative if they don't offer that option themselves. Call ahead and inquire!

Many brands like Daiya have ventured into the prepared foods arena with offerings like vegan mac and cheese and Kite Hill's vegan spinach and ricotta ravioli.

Deli

Tofurky blazed the trail in alternatives to deli sliced meats, like hickory-smoked turkey, bologna, deli ham, peppered deli slices, and more. Also, Tofurky's "Feast" is a great Thanksgiving main dish. Yves and Lightlife make many varieties of deli slices too. The gourmet company Field Roast has recently joined in and offers deli slices in flavors like smoked tomato, lentil sage, or wild mushroom.

Eggs

There are a number of egg replacers on the market. For those of you old enough to remember, Jolly Joan used to be the only brand seen at the health food store, but now Ener-G Egg Replacer has taken over that company. This product helps to leaven breads, pancakes and muffins with the aid of potato and tapioca starch. By adding this powder to water, this product can replace the use of eggs but has no nutritional value.

The new kid in town is "Follow Your Heart" Vegan Egg (packaged in traditional "egg-crate" style); a powder that can revolutionize vegan diets by reproducing the taste, texture, and properties of eggs. By combining algal (algae) flour and soybeans with black salt, the same smell and texture of eggs can be created. Served scrambled, or in omelets or vegetable quiches, the dishes created are quite delicious. Even desserts and vegetables recipes made with this product result in light and fluffy dishes, without baking soda or powder. A must-try, because it delivers flavor and consistency with some protein and has no cholesterol or sugar.

Fish

Arguably Gardein brand's "Golden Fishless Fillet" is the most popular alternative, and this company also offers mini-crabless cakes. Caroline's makes a canned "Fishless Tuna."

A newer company looking to upset the apple cart (or fish cart!) is Sophie's. With its mission to make plant-based seafood accessible and delicious to everyone, Sophie's is not kidding around. Indeed, Sophie's offers a wide range of products that includes smoked salmon, scallops, seafood Jambalaya, fish fillet, coconut shrimp, and, yes, even "toona." Newer products include salmon bacon, smoked salmon pastrami, and more!

Ice Cream

Vegan alternatives to traditional dairy ice cream are plentiful. Tofutti, one of the original purveyors of frozen desserts that include "Cuties" (ice cream sandwiches), cones, and fudgsicles, is no longer unique. From So Delicious frozen desserts to Luna & Larry's Coconut Bliss, to gourmet brands—your choices are limited only by your imagination! Or, take a trip to your local Ben & Jerry's. They now offer a number of vegan options—though we recommend healthier options like the So Delicious brand (soy, coconut, or cashew milk varieties) without those unhealthy corn syrup solids.

Meatballs

No need to let your spaghetti stand alone. Vegan meatballs to the rescue! Many brands including Gardein, Amy's, Boca, and

Morningstar, offer various flavor options. Even Trader Joe's has joined the fray with their own brand.

Milk

Today, there are many brands of organic, sweetened or unsweetened almond, coconut, rice, and soymilks available in stores. The pioneer in the field was Edensoy, and it's now joined by WestSoy, So Delicious, Pacific Natural Foods, Blue Diamond, Silk, Zen Soy, Trader Joe's, 365, among others. A newer entry into this market is Good Karma's Flax milk, providing vegans with an excellent way to get Omega 3s. It's available in various flavors and, like the Silk brand, you can find this flax milk in the dairy (or other refrigerated) section.

Looking for a vegan creamer? A variety of brands and flavors are available in liquid or powder form. Among the brands are: Califia Farms, Silk, So Delicious, SoyGo, Wildwood, and Trader Joe's.

Also, you can find numerous cookbook and online recipes that can help you make a wide variety of plant-based "milks" by blending raw nuts, seeds, and grains with water. Almonds, cashews, macadamias, Brazil nuts, hazelnuts, pecans, pistachios, coconuts, soybeans, hemp seeds, pumpkin seeds, sunflower seeds, sesame seeds, flaxseeds, quinoa, millet, rice, and oats can all be liquefied into delicious, nutritional milks.

Versatile Alternative: Tofu

Tofu, or bean curd, was one of the first foods that new vegetarians embraced when searching for alternatives to meat, fish, poultry, and eggs. Back in the day, there was usually one brand and one consistency of tofu. Today, that has all changed. So, it's important to get to know your tofu. Look for the organic label, "expire by" dates, and texture.

The extra-firm texture of tofu is great for stir-fries, kebabs, and slicing for sandwiches. Firm texture is often used for scrambles, soups, and baked goods. Silken tofu is ideal for creamy desserts, salad dressings, sauces, and the like. Baked, flavored tofu is perfect for quick fixes: add to salads, sandwiches, skillet meals; it's even yummy as a snack eaten right out of the fridge.

Some popular brands of tofu include Nasoya, Wildwood, and Mori-Nu. Wildwood's line of baked tofu includes flavors like Savory, Indian Curry, Royal Thai, or Teriyaki. Mori-Nu is a brand that features a type of silken tofu that lends itself to dips, puddings, and creamy textured recipes. While most tofu products are found in the cooler section of markets, Mori-Nu brand is sold in a unique aseptic package that protects fresh tofu from light and bacteria, allowing for a long shelf life without refrigeration—and without the use of preservatives.

Yogurt

For those of you who think that you will need to sacrifice the benefits and enjoyment of yogurt if you choose to go vegan, think again! Most of the companies who now bring us varieties of non-dairy milks and frozen desserts, also offer vegan soy, almond, and coconut yogurts. So Delicious, Kite Hill, Stonyfield, Daiya, COYO, Almond Dream, and Trader Joe's are among the many brands. Daiya even makes a Greek yogurt. Most vegan yogurt contains probiotics, which help to improve digestion, one of the reasons why dairy yogurt first became popular. Aspiring vegans, please note that not all soy yogurt is vegan as some contain casein or whey. So, be sure to read the label and look for brands clearly marked "vegan."

CHAPTER 23:

HEALTHFUL METHODS OF COOKING

There are so many opinions about the best ways to prepare one's food. After carefully choosing the types of foods that you want to eat in light of your nature, constitution, appetite, and regional food availability, you have yet one more decision to make: to cook or not to cook. Some believe that food should be eaten raw, ostensibly "heated or cooked" by the sun, thereby extracting the highest form of nutrition in its natural form.

However, it may take a physical system that is in close-to optimum condition in order to have the enzymes necessary to digest and convert these raw foods to energy. Additionally, you would need maximum chewing power for many vegetables to be able to fully digest and be integrated into your system, unless you were consuming them blended into salads or as raw juices. So that you are sure to maintain a balanced diet, we do recommend including some amount of raw food, in the form of fruits, salads, or crudités, on a daily basis if possible.

Cooked food may provide warmth and comfort to the body and can add to one's calorie load. For some people, cooked food tends to be easier to digest than its raw cousins. Recommendations for good cooking methods include, steaming, sautéing with added water, baking, broiling/oven roasting, and stir-frying with a wok—techniques that transform raw products into interesting and attractive cooked dishes.

Two methods that we don't recommend are grilling (with charcoal) and microwaved cooking. Briefly, some believe barbecuing with charcoal may be carcinogenic because of the chemicals released, including the starter fuel necessary to begin the process. These get into the food and may be harmful when ingested. Microwaving may be dangerous, as it changes the molecular nature of the foods and may damage one's blood and immune system. Perhaps it could be used sparingly to defrost a food like bread quickly, but be careful not to stand in front of the microwave when operating it.

It is recommended that leftover foods are stored in glass or stainless steel containers. Chemicals in plastic containers can leech into foods, so we don't recommend using them. Also, for the same reason, we don't recommend microwaving any food items in plastic containers. Labeling the dishes at the time of freezing helps make it easier to identify later on.

Prepared food items can be kept frozen up to three months; after three months they should be discarded.

Baking

Baking may be a slower means of getting the edibles to the table, but the process seals in the goodness of the product while allowing it to cook in its own juices. Placing the food in parchment paper (available in most stores, right next to the foils and plastic wraps) or wrapped in brown unprocessed baking paper, rather than just wrapping it in aluminum foil, is a boon to this clean cooking method. Sealing in all the nutrients, without drying out the food in the heat of the oven, this method is perfect for cooking a mélange of vegetables or soy products. It stops the browning effect that the oven creates and keeps the food warm until serving. Individual portions of delectable foods cooked with herbs and spices add a festive touch to holiday dinners.

Baking is preferable to frying vegetables—like eggplant or zucchini, for example—in recipes that require breading. Simply dip the thin slices, coat with water or the vegan egg ("Follow Your Heart") product, and dip in the breadcrumbs (preferably whole wheat); bake on a sheet that is lightly coated with spray oil. Turn when brown on one side and continue to bake until ready to assemble with sauce and vegan cheese, cover and put back into the oven to complete the cooking process.

Broiling or Oven Roasting

Broiling and oven roasting are useful methods when you want to add a browned or golden tint to the food, but they must be used carefully. These methods are best done with a dish that's already been cooked or for garlic bread that needs to have a few minutes of top browning to finish off the presentation. Since the temperature from the top coil is so high (400–550 degrees), the food can easily burn, so keep the oven light on in order to observe the process and know when the dish is done. Roasted root veggies are a great winter favorite and are usually tossed and coated with a small amount of oil and baked in a 400-degree oven on the lower rack for about 40 minutes. Top browning can be done with moving the dish to the upper rack and turning the oven to broil to get that brown toasted finish.

Sauteing

Today, with our more health-conscious population, one of the increasingly popular methods is sautéing. Sauté the ingredients with a slight spray of olive or sunflower oil until the food sizzles and then add a small amount of pure water, actually creating a little steaming effect. Sautéing cooks the food up quickly without using a lot of oil. Remember to stir the pan and add more water if needed. Fried and deep-fried foods should be avoided as the absorption of too much oil saturating the vegetable is not good for the body. Some suggest heating the oil first until it's warm before putting the vegetable in the pan.

Steaming

The use of a stainless-steel pot or bamboo steamer basket inside a stainless steel (not aluminum) pot is one of the best and easiest methods for cooking vegetables and tofu. Valuable minerals are not lost, as happens with boiling or overcooking. Add water to the level just below the steamer basket and cook over a medium flame with a tight cover on. The usual rule of thumb: try to cook the food until it is at the height of its bright color and stop just before it fades in order to get the maximum nutrient value. That should also indicate the necessary time to make the vegetable tender, which just takes a few minutes. Make sure that the water does not cook out by checking it and replenishing with more water, if necessary, throughout the process. Any water remaining is valuable, and you can save it in a glass jar and refrigerate it to use for broths, for future sauces, for gravies, and to add to soups. It contains many of the beneficial vitamins that have been leached throughout the steaming, although hopefully just a minimum amount is lost.

Stir Frying

The Chinese have mastered this art. They invented the stainless-steel wok, which has the perfect contour for cooking leftover rice, tofu, and vegetables evenly and quickly. Follow the instructions to season a new wok, but if you already have been using the wok for years, the coating should be ready to go. Never use abrasives to clean the wok but use just a little dish soap and water. Then, dry the wok on the stove for one to two minutes before storing it. How we treat our equipment creates a vibration for the food and for the diner. Try to create *sattvic* (pure) energy by handling items in the kitchen with kindness and care.

To stir fry: prepare ginger root (if desired), vegetables, and other ingredients and lay them out on your cutting board close to the pan. Use high-heat tolerant oil, like sunflower, and heat the pan first. Then add the oil until it sizzles. Start with the densest ingredients first (like carrots or broccoli) first, as they require the longest cooking time. As you stir, add each ingredient in the order of its texture or tenderness. Mung bean or other sprouts should be added last as they contain mostly water and cook quickly. Add a little water to the wok if necessary in order to keep it all moving or to generate a base for a sauce that you might like to create. This method of "flash-cooking" helps to seal in the deliciousness of the flavors and blends the spices together. Add some seasonings like tamari or toasted sesame oil at the end for the finale.

PART VI:

RESOURCES

CHAPTER 24:
ORGANIZATIONS

From the Vegetarian Society founded in England in 1847, to the American Vegan Society—the world's first vegan organization—there are numerous organizations that exist solely to advocate for vegetarianism/veganism, to provide information, and to organize events.

American Vegan Society: www.americanvegan.org

Provides fact sheets on topics including nutrition and health.

Farm Sanctuary: www.farmsanctuary.org

Farm Sanctuary's mission is to protect farm animals from cruelty, inspire change in the way society views and treats farm animals, and promote compassionate vegan living.

International Vegetarian Union: www.ivu.org

IVU links the majority of societies and associations around the world. Sponsors annual congresses that feature speakers and workshops on the subjects of vegetarianism and health.

North American Vegetarian Society: www.navs-online.org

A dual mission: to provide a support network and to inform the public about how vegetarianism benefits humans, other animals, and the earth. Each year, NAVS sponsors World Vegetarian Day (October 1st) celebrations around the country: www.worldvegetarianday.org.

People for the Ethical Treatment of Animals: www.peta.org

The largest animal rights organization in the world, with more than 5 million members and supporters.

Physician's Committee on Responsible Medicine: www.pcrm.org

Founded by Dr. Neil Barnard, PCRM does a great deal of advocacy work and promotes a vegan lifestyle.

Toronto Vegetarian Society: www.veg.ca

Has a mission to inspire people to choose a healthier, greener, more compassionate lifestyle through plant-based eating.

Vegan Society: www.vegansociety.com

Provides fact sheets on vegan topics including nutrition and health.

Vegetarian Resource Group: www.vrg.org

Offers numerous resources, including listings of restaurants in the US and Canada.

Vegetarian Society: www.vegsoc.org

Offers membership, as well as an online community and resources, for example, an online guide for new vegetarians.

Vegetarian Society of DC: www.vsdc.org

An educational nonprofit promoting the benefits of vegetarianism through education, community-building, and social activities.

VegSource: www.vegsource.com

Vegetarian/vegan recipes, discussion boards, articles, information from medical doctors, experts and nutritionists, and an online community.

CHAPTER 25:

WEBSITES

In addition to the websites for the organizations listed in Chapter 24, there are many more websites dedicated to providing resources for vegetarians and vegans. Here is a sampling of some of the best.

Go Dairy Free: www.godairyfree.org

How to cook, shop, and dine dairy free with special emphasis on vegan diets.

GoVeg.com

How to go vegan in 3 easy steps.

Jazzy Vegetarian: www.jazzyvegetarian.com

Laura Theodore's website. She also hosts the Jazzy Vegetarian vegan cooking series on public television and the Jazzy Vegetarian Radio podcast.

Savvy Vegetarian: www.savvyvegetarian.com

Support for vegetarian/vegan lifestyle featuring life coaching, courses, educational articles, reviews, recipes and resource guide.

Vegan.com: www.vegan.com

A website dedicated to making the transition to vegan diet and all things vegan. A massive array of resources from news to recipes to product reviews and more.

Vegan Feed: veganfeed.com

Exhaustive index of links—organized by themes—to articles, recipes, videos, and podcasts on vegan lifestyle.

Vegan Street: www.veganstreet.com

A major source of vegan tools, resources, community and culture.

Vegan Village: www.veganvillage.co.uk

Initially created to promote vegan companies online and links to around 200 vegan companies and contacts in the UK.

Vegetarian Site: www.thevegetariansite.com

Online portal for vegan living. Sections include animal rights, health and nutrition, news, editorials, free recipes, cruelty-free shopping, events.

VegFamily: www.vegfamily.com

A great resource for vegan family living, including pregnancy information, parenting advice, travel guides, and product reviews.

Veggie Global: www.veggieglobal.com

An abundance of resources ranging from nutritional guidance, environmental impact information, animal rights, and activist campaigns.

CHAPTER 26:
PUBLICATIONS AND VIDEOS

There are more and more books published every day on the subject of vegetarian and vegan cooking and lifestyle. There are also more and more films and videos made about veg lifestyle, healthy eating, and animal rights. In addition to the many veg journals and magazines published, most of the organizations and websites in Chapters 24 and 25 offer free newsletters. For those just transitioning to veg diets or for those hoping to inspire others to make the switch, vegetarian starter kits are a wonderful aid. Here is just a small sampling and selection of some of the best of these resources to date.

Books-General

The China Study by T. Colin Campbell, Ph.D.
and Thomas M. Campbell II

Crazy Sexy Diet by Kris Carr

Diet for a New Planet and The Food Revolution by John Robbins

Eating Animals by Jonathan Safran Foer

How Not to Die by Michael Greger, M.D.

The Kind Diet by Alicia Silverstone

Stress, Diet and Your Heart by Dean Ornish, M.D.

The Veganist by Kathy Freston

The World Peace Diet by Will Tuttle, Ph.D.

Yoga and Vegetarianism by Sharon Gannon

Books-Children's

Apples, Bean Dip, and Carrot Cake: Kids! Teach Yourself to Cook
by Anne and Freya Dinshah (for ages 4–12)

Saving Emily by Nicholas Read (for ages 10 and up)

Vegan is Love by Ruby Roth (for ages 7 and up)

Cookbooks

1000 Vegan Recipes by Robin Robertson

The Back to Eden Cookbook by Jethro Kloss

The Candle Cafe Cookbook by Pierson and Potenza

Crazy Sexy Kitchen by Kris Carr

The Get Healthy, Go Vegan Cookbook by Neal Barnard, MD

More Great Good Dairy-free Desserts (Naturally)
by Fran Costigan

The New Vegan by Áine Carlin

Professional Vegetarian Cooking by Ken Bergeron

Simple Recipes for Joy by Sharon Gannon

Ten Talents by Frank and Rosalie Hurd

DVDs

Blackfish

Cowspiracy

Eating (3rd Ed.)

Fed Up?

Food Inc.

Food Matters

Forks Over Knives

Peaceable Kingdom

Vegucated

Journals

American Vegan: www.americanvegan.org
Quarterly publication from the American Vegan Society

Vegetarian Journal: www.vrg.org
Quartlery publication of the Vegetarian Resource Group

Vegetarian Voice: www.navs-online.org
Published by North American Vegetarian Society

VegNews: VegNews.com
Great vegan recipes sent every week for free

Vegan Travel Guides

The Essential Vegan Travel Guide by Caitlin Galer Unti

Vegetarian Travel with Happy Cow: www.happycow.net

Vegetarian and Vegan Travel Guide: circleourearth.com

Vegan Travel Guide: www.angloitalianfollowus.com

Vegan Travel Supporting Vegans Worldwide: www.vegantravel.com

Vegetarian Starter Kits

Some organizations offer these for free download and some offer printed copies. You can also purchase larger quantities, which are great for sharing with friends or distributing at gatherings.

Animals Australia: whyveg.com/kit

Going Veggie—What to Eat: issuu.com/vegsoc

Farm Sanctuary: farmsanctuary.org/learn/educational-literature

Mercy for Animals: chooseveg.com/vsg

PETA: peta.org/living/food/free-vegan-starter-kit/free-vegan-starter-kit-friend

Physician's Committee for Responsible Medicine: pcrm.org/health/diets/vsk

PART VII:

RECIPES

CHAPTER 27:

SEVEN DAYS OF HEALTHY MEALS

Below is a list of suggested meal choices for you to mix and match depending on your appetite and constitution, which varies from day to day. It includes a variety of different grains, nuts, seeds, and vegetables, plus soups and salads to tease your taste buds and delight your tummy! Note that fresh fruit can be eaten if desired with any of the meals, avoiding melons, which should be consumed separately. In order to make any dish gluten-free, substitute Bob's Red Mill gluten-free flour blends or pancake mixes. All recipes are free of any animal products. Make sure you include at least one fresh salad in each day's mix and match selection for optimum health.

Breakfasts

1. Very Vegan Omelet
2. Super Soy French Toast
3. Glorious Granola
4. Tasty Tofu Scramble
5. Best Blueberry Pancakes
6. Quinoa Cooked Cereal with Berries & Nuts
7. Bountiful Banana Bread

Lunches

1. Brown Rice and Lentil Soup
2. Quinoa & Bean Salad
3. Tempting Tofu Mini Quiches
4. Classy Chopped Greens & Arugula Salad with Dressing + Guacamole & Tortilla Chips
5. Bold Broccoli Soup with Greens + Crackers
6. Cold Sesame Noodles over Spinach
7. Tabouli Salad, Baba Ghanoush, & Whole Wheat Pita Bread

Dinners

1. Pesto with Pizazz + Side Salad
2. Savory Seitan Stew + Thai Peanut Spinach
3. Couscous and Lentil Pilaf + Veggie Dish + Raisin Chutney
4. Soba Noodles with Vegetables in Miso Sauce
5. Pilau Rice with Mung dal + Side of Yogurt
6. Vegetable Stroganoff
7. Hearty Minestrone Soup + Whole Grain Bread

Desserts

1. Rice Crispy Cashew Treats
2. Miniature Peanut Butter and Jelly Cookies
3. Tofu Almond Cream with Fresh Fruit
4. Ginger Carrot Cake

5. Rice Pudding
6. Outrageous Oatmeal Cookies
7. Divine Date-Nut Treats

Quick Fixes & Kid Friendly Mini-meals and Snacks

1. Veggie Burgers on Whole Wheat Bun + Sweet Potato Fries
2. Mock Turkey Sandwiches on Whole Grain Bread
3. Tofu Dogs on Whole Grain Buns + Rosemary Potatoes
4. Mock Tuna Salad on Whole Grain Bread
   with Cherry Tomatoes & Carrot Sticks
5. Gardein Crispy "Chicken" Tenders
6. Seasoned Organic Popcorn
7. Frozen Desserts & Fruits

BREAKFAST RECIPES

1. Very Vegan Omelet

Yields 2 hearty-sized portions

Combine:

½ cup	rice flour
½ cup	whole wheat pastry flour
1 cup	coconut milk ("So Delicious Culinary-lite")
½ cup	water
2 Tbs.	nutritional yeast
2 tsp.	turmeric powder
½ tsp.	sea salt (or try black salt which adds an eggy taste)

In a large skillet, sauté in 1 Tbs. oil (extra virgin olive or sunflower oil) diced pieces of:

½ cup	red pepper
½ cup	green pepper
½ cup	white or yellow onion
1	small scallion
4	sliced mushrooms (add last)

Reserve:

½ cup	cheddar vegan cheese (Daiya or Follow your Heart shredded cheddar)
½ cup	organic tomato sauce fresh organic salsa to taste

1. It is best to use a non-stick skillet for this recipe. Stir veggies until onion is translucent about 5 minutes and mushrooms start to produce liquid. Remove from frying pan and set aside.

2. Rinse pan if residue remains and spray a small amount of oil and heat again to medium. Mix omelet batter again, making sure it is quite thin and pour one ladle at a time about half the batter. Quickly tilt the pan before it is set to create an even layer of batter. It should be set in about 3 min.

3. Then add half the cooked veggies and ¼ cup grated vegan cheese per omelet into the center, quickly flip and fold in half and allow to cook 1 minute more. Can be turned over with a spatula and browned on both sides or removed at this point.

4. This can be served with heated tomato sauce on top (¼ cup per serving) and topped with fresh parsley sprig. Also tasty with fresh salsa on the side. Add peas to the vegetables for a "Spanish" version. Whole wheat or rye toast is a good complement to this dish.

2. Super Soy French Toast

Serves 2–3

1 cup	soft silken tofu (low fat)
¾ cup	vanilla soymilk
1 tsp.	vanilla alcohol-free extract
½ tsp.	maple syrup or agave nectar
¼ tsp.	ground cinnamon
¼ cup	fresh squeezed orange juice
8	slices whole grain bread or rolls
	sunflower oil spray

1. Mix all ingredients in a food processor until smooth and well combined. Pour the mixture into a large shallow bowl.

2. Dip the bread into the mixture, coating both sides generously, and fry in a medium hot skillet that has been lightly sprayed with oil. Add more cinnamon sprinkled on top before frying to taste.

3. Cook and turn over until slightly brown on both sides, about 5 minutes.

Serve with maple syrup. If necessary, the leftover batter can be refrigerated for future use within 1–2 days.

Optional: Serve with cooked vegetarian bacon strips on the side.

3. Glorious Granola

This recipe is a wholesome mixture of grains, nuts, seeds and fruit that is an excellent breakfast cereal, as well as, a delicious topping for cooked grain cereals and apple pie.

3 cups	organic rolled oats
¼ cup	wheat germ (omit for gluten-free)
¼ cup	hemp seeds
¼ cup	sesame seeds (raw)
¼ cup	sunflower seeds (raw and unsalted)
½ cup	walnuts chopped
½ cup	pecans chopped
½ cup	cashews: some chopped, some whole
¼ cup	peanuts or almonds (slivered)
¼ cup	coconut flakes
1 tsp.	cinnamon

Mix well, set aside.

½ cup	raisins or currants
½ cup	dried cranberries, sweet and plump
¼ cup	goji berries (optional)
1 tsp.	cinnamon

Mix well and reserve.

In a saucepan, combine over medium heat:

½ cup	pure maple sugar syrup
½ cup	light agave syrup
2 tsp.	vanilla alcohol-free extract
½ cup	sunflower oil or water if oil-free

Heat for a few minutes, just until boil, stirring occasionally.

1. Pour the heated sweet liquid over the oat mixture and mix well.

2. Spray 2 large baking pans with sunflower oil and spread the mixtures evenly on both pans, in one layer.

3. Bake at 325 degrees for about 20–25 minutes, stirring away from the sides every 10 minutes to prevent uneven browning.

4. Bake until golden brown. Remove and pour into a big bowl to cool.

5. When cool add the unbaked raisin mixture to the oats and nuts and mix well. (Note: this method keeps the dried fruit moist and fresh tasting and is a contrast to the toasted flavor of the granola).

6. Store in glass jars with tight lids in the pantry.

Excellent with soy- or nut-based milks or with plant-based yogurts like coconut and almond varieties!

4. Tasty Tofu Scramble

Yields 2–3 hearty servings

1	package 14 ounce "lite" firm tofu
6	strips "Smart Bacon" by Lightlife
	(optional; adds 12 more grams of protein)
¾ cup	white onion diced
2	scallions chopped
½ cup	green pepper
1 cup	mushrooms sliced thinly (any variety)
1 Tbs.	tamari (low-sodium if possible) or more to taste
½ cup	shredded non-dairy cheese
	(Daiya mozzarella or cheddar flavor)
1 tsp.	turmeric
	sunflower spray oil (to lightly cover the frying pan)

1. Rinse the tofu with fresh water and cut into about 4 slices lengthwise. Drain well with paper towels or cheesecloth, pressing out most of the moisture. Set aside.

2. Separate the bacon strips, dice and fry in a light spray of oil until just starting to brown.

3. Add the chopped veggies and cook for a few minutes while stirring.

4. Crumble the tofu into small chunks and add to pan.

5. Stir and add the tamari and turmeric (note, the yellow color will emerge as you cook the tofu longer).

6. When heated throughout, add the cheese shreds and stir until melted.

Serve with whole grain bread or sprouted English muffins.

5. Best Blueberry Pancakes

Yields 8 medium-size pancakes

Bob's Red Mill Brand "7 Grain" Pancake and Waffle mix is one of the best vegan mixes on the market. They also carry a gluten-free pancake mix that is quite flavorful.

1¼ cups	pancake mix
1 Tbs.	sunflower oil
¾ cup	any plant-based cold "milk"
1 tsp.	vanilla extract (non-alcohol)
½ tsp.	cinnamon
½ cup	fresh blueberries. Some prefer added to wet mixture before grilling or reserved for topping on cooked pancakes.

Optional: 1 egg substitute (either use Follow your Heart Vegan Egg or Ener-G brand for fluffier pancakes)—but also can be omitted and still comes out fine!

1. Mix ingredients well just until blended. Do not over mix. Add blueberries now if desired inside the pancakes and blend gently.

2. Use spray oil to coat the griddle lightly. Heat on medium setting 1–2 minutes.

3. Pour about ¼ cup mixture when grill is hot and cook, turning once when edges start to brown and bubbles are in the center. Note: the blueberries, if inside, may start to ooze when close to ready.

Serve with the reserved blueberries on top and pure maple syrup, or other sweetened liquid.

6. Quinoa Cooked Cereal (with berries and nuts)

Serves 2

1 cup	organic flax, nut, or soy milk
1 cup	water
1 cup	organic quinoa, rinsed well
1 cup	fresh organic blackberries
1 cup	fresh organic raspberries
½ tsp.	ground cinnamon
⅓ cup	chopped walnuts or almonds, toasted*
4 tsp.	organic agave nectar or 4–5 drops of liquid stevia to taste (try vanilla creme flavor)

1. Combine milk, water, and quinoa in a medium saucepan.

2. Bring to a boil over high heat. Reduce heat to medium-low; cover and simmer 15 minutes or until most of the liquid is absorbed.

3. Turn off heat; let stand covered for 5 minutes.

4. Stir in blackberries, raspberries, and cinnamon, as well as stevia (if using that).

5. Transfer to four bowls and top with pecans.

6. Drizzle 1 teaspoon agave nectar over each serving (if not using stevia).

*While the quinoa cooks, roast the walnuts in a toaster oven at 350 degrees for 5 to 6 minutes

7. Bountiful Banana Bread

2	large very ripe bananas
2 cups	whole wheat flour
½ cup	applesauce
½ cup	soy, flax, or almond milk
1 Tbs.	baking soda
1 tsp.	ground pumpkin spice blend
1 tsp.	ground cinnamon
¼ cup	raisins
¼ cup	fresh blueberries
dash	ground ginger
	salt & stevia to taste (optional)

Preheat oven to 350 degrees.

1. Place the flour in a large mixing bowl. Add in the baking soda and mix thoroughly. Add spices (and salt, from a pinch to whatever desired). Set aside.

2. Place the bananas in another bowl and mash well. Add in the applesauce and "milk" and stir well until evenly mixed.

3. Combine both bowls of ingredients into one and stir well. Then, add raisins, blueberries, chocolate chips (if desired) and mix.

4. Coat a 9-inch loaf pan with oil (or spray with canola oil spray). Pour mixture into the pan.

5. Place in oven and bake for 75 minutes.

6. Once baking is complete, remove pan from the oven and let sit for 15 minutes.

7. Then, remove the bread from the pan (easily done by placing a plate over the pan, then, using potholders, so you don't get burned, turn the plate and pan over and the bread will slide out.) Carefully pick up bread and place on a wire rack to cool.

Serve with tofu cream cheese.

LUNCH RECIPES

1. Brown Rice and Lentil Soup

Serves 4

½ cup	long grain brown rice
½ cup	red lentils
½ cup	fresh peas, shelled
1	onion, finely chopped
2	cloves garlic, crushed
1 Tbs.	sunflower oil
4 cups	vegetable stock
1 tsp.	ground coriander
¼ tsp.	ground cinnamon
¼ tsp.	ground cardamom
	fresh parsley
	black pepper to taste

1. Warm the oil and gently sauté onion and garlic.

2. Mix in spices and stir for one minute more.

3. Add all other ingredients except peas and parsley; bring to a boil.

4. Cover and simmer about 25 minutes, stirring occasionally, until rice and lentils are cooked.

5. Add peas and mix until they are warmed through.

6. Garnish with parsley.

2. Quinoa and Black Bean Salad (with Orange Dressing)

Serves 4–6

1	cup	uncooked quinoa (any color), rinsed, and drained
2	cups	water
2		large oranges
¼	cup	extra virgin olive oil
2	tsp.	apple cider vinegar
½	tsp.	agave nectar
½	tsp.	coriander seeds, toasted and lightly crushed
½	tsp.	salt
¼	cup	chopped cilantro
1½	cups*	cooked black beans, rinsed and drained
½		small red onion, thinly sliced
		freshly ground black pepper to taste

1. Place quinoa and water in a small saucepan. Bring to a boil, cover, and simmer over low heat. Simmer for about 15 minutes, or until all liquid is absorbed.

2. Remove from heat and let stand for 5 minutes. Fluff quinoa with a fork and spread on a parchment-lined baking sheet to cool.

3. Prepare oranges while quinoa is cooling. Finely grate the zest (skin) of one orange and set aside. Separate both oranges into segments, reserving the juice (squeezing the orange membranes after segmenting), and set aside.

4. In a small bowl, whisk together orange zest, 3 tablespoons of orange juice, olive oil, apple cider vinegar, agave, coriander seeds, salt, a few turns of pepper, and chopped cilantro.

Adjust seasonings if desired.

5. Place quinoa, black beans, onion, and orange segments in a large bowl and stir gently to combine. Pour dressing over salad and toss gently to coat.

Serve immediately or refrigerate until ready to serve.

* Or, you can use one whole can of the beans

3. Tempting Tofu Mini Quiches

Serves 3–4

1 tsp.	minced garlic
½ cup	green pepper, chop finely
1 cup	mushrooms (white or Baby Bella), chop finely:
¼ cup	fresh chives, chop finely or 1 scallion
	black pepper to taste
	olive oil spray

In a food processor combine the following:

12-oz.	package of Mori-Nu lite silken firm tofu (water drained)
¼ cup	plain soymilk
2 Tbs.	nutritional yeast
1 Tbs.	arrowroot powder
1 tsp.	tahini (sesame paste)
¼ tsp.	onion powder
¼ tsp.	turmeric
½ tsp.	sea salt
½ tsp.	black salt (imparts an eggy flavor)

1. Preheat oven to 375 degrees. Spray muffin tins with olive oil.

2. Lightly spray a skillet with the olive oil and sauté the veggies, and black pepper until the liquid just starts to come out. Set aside.

3. Once what you put in the food processor is completely smooth, you can add the tofu mixture to the sautéed veggies and combine well.

4. Spoon the mixture into each muffin tin about halfway full. Put into oven and quickly turn down to 350 degrees.

5. Bake about 30 minutes depending on the type of tins used and your individual oven. They are ready when an inserted toothpick comes out clean.

6. Remove from oven and let cool about 10 minutes before removing carefully from the pan.

These can be enjoyed room temperature or slightly reheated if prepared ahead of time. They are gluten free and high in protein. The type of veggies used are subject to your imagination so be creative but conservative as too much volume might affect the ability of the mixture to hold together.

4. Classy Chopped Greens and Arugula Salad with Dressing & Guacamole + Tortilla Chips

Salad
Serves 6

1	basket cherry tomatoes, halved
1	fennel bulb, stalks trimmed, thinly sliced
1	cucumber, seeded and diced
1	sweet bell pepper, seeded and diced
1	bunch arugula, chopped
1	avocado, peeled and chopped in cubes
	juice of 1–2 lemons
	salt and pepper

1. Prepare all vegetables, mix and toss with lemon juice, olive oil, and salt and pepper to taste.

2. Don't be afraid to over dress the salad. With its peppery taste and tough leaf, arugula really needs a lot of dressing and some salt too.

Amazing Almond Dressing
(Yogaville's most requested recipe!): Yields about 1/2 quart

½ cup	raw, unsalted almonds
½ cup	nutritional yeast
½ cup	safflower oil
½ cup	water
¼ cup	tamari

1. Using a high-power food processor, blend all the ingredients until creamy.

172

2. Add water to adjust consistency.

3. Savory uses for all seasons: Get creative! Try it as a dressing for a cold buckwheat noodle salad in the summer or as a marinade for baked tofu in the fall.

Una Bella Guacamole
Serves 4

2	ripe avocados
2 Tbs.	red onion, minced
½	cucumber peeled and diced finely
1–2	chopped roma tomatoes
1	large garlic clove
¼ cup	cilantro leaves
2 pinches	cayenne
	juice of 1 or 2 limes
	salt to taste

1. Chop onion and garlic until finely minced.

2. Chop cilantro separately until also minced super-fine.

3. Mash avocados gently, mix in other ingredients, spices, and lime juice to taste.

5. Bold Broccoli Soup with Greens + Crackers

Broccoli soup

Serves 8

1½	bunches broccoli
¼ cup	olive oil
1	large garlic clove, minced
½ cup	chopped yellow onion
½	bunch of greens, chopped coarsely
1 Tbs.	dried basil
1 Tbs.	mustard seeds
6 cups	water
	juice of ½ lemon
	salt
	pepper

1. Divide the broccoli into florets of equal size, 2 to 3 inches long. Trim the stalks by cutting off the ends and peeling off the thick skin with a paring knife.

2. Slice all the parts into bite-size pieces. Set aside 1 cup of florets for adding later.

3. Heat oil in a large pot, add the garlic and onion and cook over high heat, stirring frequently for 3–4 minutes until the onion is translucent.

4. Stir in the herbs and mustard seeds.

5. Continue to cook for 1 minute, then toss in the broccoli (reserving the 1 cup of florets) and cook for 2–3 minutes stirring continually.

6. Add the water and bring to a simmer. Cover and cook for 1 hour.

7. Puree the soup in a food processor or with a hand blender. Thin it with more water if necessary.

8. Return to the stove and stir in the remaining florets and the chopped greens.

9. Add the lemon juice, salt, and pepper to taste.

10. Cook over low heat until the florets are bright green and tender yet crunchy and the greens are wilted.

Serve with your choice of whole-grain crackers.

6. Cold Sesame Noodles over Spinach

Serves 4–6

12 oz	whole wheat or buckwheat noodles
1½ Tbs.	finely grated fresh ginger
1½ Tbs.	finely grated daikon radish
1 Tbs.	tahini
1½ Tbs.	toasted sesame oil
4 Tbs.	tamari
4–5 Tbs.	water
1½ Tbs.	fresh lemon juice
½	red or green pepper, cored seeded and cut into slivers, to garnish
3 Tbs.	toasted sesame seeds
1	bunch of spinach, washed, and trimmed

1. Cook noodles in boiling water until tender but still firm.

2. Drain thoroughly and rinse with cold water, then chill in the refrigerator for at least one hour.

3. With the exception of the spinach and pepper garnish, whisk the remaining ingredients together in a bowl and leave to stand for a few minutes.

4. Pour dressing over the noodles and toss well just before serving.

5. Garnish with pepper and sesame seeds.

Serve on a platter over a bed of fresh spinach.

7. Tabouli Salad, Baba Ghanoush + Whole Wheat Pita Bread

Tabouli Salad

Yields 8 cups

2	cups	bulgur
3¼	cups	water
1	tsp.	Spike seasoning (to taste)
¾	cup	lime juice
½	Tbs.	minced garlic
¼	cup	olive oil (or more, as desired)
¼	cup	mint
¼	cup	chopped green onions
1½	cups	cherry tomatoes, cut in ½ or ¼
1	cup	chopped fresh parsley
1	cup	shredded carrot
½		skinned and seeded cucumbers
2		diced medium yellow summer squash (optional)
		salt and pepper to taste

1. Boil water with the Spike in a pot, remove from stove, and add the bulgur and summer squash.

2. Let sit for 20 minutes, and then put in the refrigerator to cool.

3. Mix in the rest of the ingredients.

Serve cold.

Baba Ghanoush

Serves 6

2	medium-small eggplants
½ cup	tahini
3	medium cloves of garlic, crushed
½ cup	finely chopped parsley
¼ cup	fine chopped scallions (optional)
1 Tbs.	olive oil
1 tsp.	salt (to taste)
	fresh ground black pepper
	juice of 1 large lemon

1. Preheat oven to 400 degrees.

2. Cut off the stem ends of the eggplants and prick them all over with a fork.

3. Place them directly on an oven rack and let them roast slowly until completely charred (about 45 minutes). When they are wrinkled, crumpled and totally soft, you'll know they are ready.

4. Remove eggplants gingerly from the oven and wait until cool enough to handle.

5. Scoop out the insides and transfer them to a food processor.

6. Pulse with remaining ingredients, except olive oil.

Chill and serve drizzled with olive oil.

DINNER RECIPES

---

1. Pesto with Pizazz, Side Salad & Dressing

Pesto with Pizazz
Serves 4

3 cups	fresh basil (trim the tough stems off and discard or use for soup)
5	medium peeled garlic cloves (or to taste)
¼ cup	raw pine nuts
½ cup	walnuts
¼ cup	virgin olive oil
¼ cup	vegan grated soy or rice topping, parmesan flavor

1. In a food processor, pulse the nuts, garlic, oil, basil, and the grated cheese—in that order—stopping occasionally to stir down the basil leaves. Pulse a few times with each addition until the nuts are quite well chopped, but still have some texture and the basil is well incorporated into an almost creamy texture.

2. Refrigerate.

3. Put into small containers (stainless steel if available) and freeze if not consumed within a few days.

Some other additions and suggestions are as follows:

1. Add some fresh spinach to the basil (some say it helps to keep the pesto greener in color).

2. Add nutritional yeast, 1–2 tablespoons of light white miso, and or 1 tablespoon of fresh lemon juice.

3. A great pesto variation utilizes fresh cilantro, onions or scallions, olive oil, walnuts, and a dash of salt.

Be creative and serve on whole wheat pasta, Asian noodles, or brown rice. This recipe can also be used with crackers, in soups, stuffed in endive leaves, and celery stalks.

Side Salad

Salads don't need to be the dull or boring side dishes we associate with fast food restaurants—iceberg lettuce (which contains almost zero nutrients), tomatoes, and cucumber. Instead, experiment with the many different types of greens that provide fresh nutrients and delicious flavors.

1. Utilize a base of organic romaine lettuce and spinach and build on it, utilizing exotic greens such as frisee, arugula, radicchio, baby beet greens, mache, baby kale, and many others. Most grocery stores even carry pre-washed organic versions in containers for easy prep as well as already prepared mixtures of various organic greens.

2. Add in alfalfa or other sprouts

3. Add organic carrots, cherry tomatoes, cucumbers, avocado, and any other veggies

Hollyhock Dressing

Yields about 1/2 a quart

This light dressing is a savory twist on the traditional oil-and-vinegar dressing.

⅓ cup	tamari
⅓ cup	balsamic vinegar
⅓ cup	water
1 cup	olive oil
1 cup	nutritional yeast

1. Blend all the ingredients until an even consistency is reached.
2. Chill (if desired)

2. Savory Seitan Stew & & Thai Peanut Spinach

Savory Seitan Stew

1	package of seitan (original or flavored), thinly sliced
2–3	carrots, sliced medium
2–3	celery stalks, sliced
2	medium white potatoes, peeled, and cubed
1	large white onion, diced or sliced
¼ cup	dried parsley
¼ cup	dried basil
2–3	small cloves of garlic, pressed or chopped fine
1	package of vegan powdered vegetable gravy (Hain brand—either mock-chicken flavored or brown gravy mix). Since this contains abundant salt do not add additional tamari.
1 cup	frozen peas (optional)

1. Put all the veggies and spices in a covered pot with a little spray oil. Sauté, adding ½ cup water to the pot, letting it steam until almost fork soft. Check for sticking and add more water if needed.

2. Add the seitan slices and if it came in a liquid, add that too.

3. Cook over low heat for about 5 minutes.

4. Add the packet of gravy and stir, then add one cup of water or more according to how thick you want the stew to be.

5. Add frozen peas if desired. Cook for about 5 minutes more.

Serve over whole grain rice or thick whole grain, soy, or bean noodles.

Thai Peanut Spinach

Serves 4

2 Tbs.	sesame oil
1	clove garlic
24 oz.	fresh spinach, washed and dried
1	lemon
½ cup	Thai Peanut Sauce (see recipe)
4 tsp.	sesame seeds, toasted

1. Sauté garlic until pale, tan, and toasted.

2. Add spinach and a little water; cook until spinach wilts.

3. Squeeze lemon juice over spinach and add Thai Peanut Sauce.

4. Sprinkle with sesame seeds.

Thai Peanut Sauce

Yields about 1½ cups

2 Tbs.	peanut butter
⅓ cup	onion, coarsely chopped
1	clove garlic, minced
¾ cup	coconut milk
½ tsp.	tamari
1 tsp.	lime juice
1 pinch	red pepper flakes
½ tsp.	fresh ginger, minced
½ tsp.	ground coriander

1. Blend all ingredients in blender or food processor until it forms a smooth paste.

2. Simmer about 10 minutes while stirring constantly.

3. Couscous and Lentil Pilaf with Veggie Side Dish & Raisin Chutney

Lentil Pilaf

Serves 4

½	cup	dried lentils
1½	cups	water
2	Tbs.	sunflower oil
1		garlic clove, minced
1	Tbs.	fresh ginger, grated
1	Tbs.	curry powder
1	pinch	cayenne
½	cup	orange juice
1	tsp.	sea salt
1	cup	peeled and diced carrots
2	cups	spinach, chopped
½	cup	scallions, chopped
1½	cups	quick-cooking couscous
1½	cups	boiling water
		salt and pepper to taste

1. Bring lentils and water to a boil, cover, and simmer over low heat, until lentils are tender (about 35 minutes). Add more water if needed.

2. While lentils are cooking, heat oil in a medium saucepan over low heat. Add the garlic, ginger, curry powder, and cayenne. Sauté for 1 minute, stirring constantly.

3. Add orange juice, salt, and carrots. Increase heat and simmer until carrots are tender, about 5 minutes.

4. Add spinach and cover for 1 minute, until spinach wilts.

5. Add scallions, couscous, boiling water and cook for 1 minute,

stirring constantly. Cover, remove from heat, and let stand for 5 minutes.

6. Fluff couscous with a fork.

7. When lentils are tender, drain and add to the mixture.

8. Add salt and pepper to taste

Serve hot. A side dish of your choice of steamed, roasted, or sautéed veggies and a side dish of yogurt or sour cream (vegan or dairy) can be added.

Raisin Chutney

Yields 1 cup (about 4 servings)

1 cup	organic raisins, plumped in a little hot water for 10 minutes
1 Tbs.	chopped fresh ginger
¼ tsp.	cayenne
½ tsp.	sea salt
¼ cup	water
	juice of ½ a lemon

1. Drain raisins, saving the water.*

2. In a blender or food processor blend raisins, ginger, cayenne, salt, and lemon juice to form a coarse paste—adding water a little bit at a time to incorporate (you may not need to use all of the water).

3. Adjust seasoning as needed. If the chutney is too spicy, add a touch more salt or lemon juice to tone it down.

4. Add more water only as a last resort; adding water will significantly thin the chutney.

*This water becomes rich with iron and other nutritious minerals—you can drink it for strength and vitality!

4. Soba Noodles with Vegetables in Miso Sauce

Serves 4

½ cup	white miso
1¼ cups	water
1	bunch basil
4	carrots
1	bunch spinach
2 cups	green beans
1	red bell pepper
3 cups	mung bean sprouts
3 Tbs.	sunflower oil
1½ lbs.	soba noodles or Explore Asian's Edamame Pasta

1. Put on a large pot of water to boil for the noodles.

2. Wash vegetables, grate carrots, chop spinach, slice pepper thinly, trim green beans, and pick basil leaves off stems.

3. Dissolve miso in 1¼ cup water.

4. Once water has boiled, add the noodles and wait until water returns to boil. Cook until noodles are just slightly firm to the bite, about 12 minutes.

5. Meanwhile, heat oil in a large pan (big enough to accommodate vegetables and noodles.)

6. Add all vegetables except sprouts, sauté five minutes; add sprouts and heat 2 minutes more.

7. Once noodles are cooked, drain, and then mix into cooked vegetables.

8. Combine with miso sauce and stir thoroughly.

Other seasonal vegetables can be substituted, with cooking times varied according to their density.

5. Pilau Rice with Mung Dal + Side of Yogurt

Pilau rice

Serves 4

2½	cups	uncooked brown basmati rice
4	cups	water
1		onion, finely chopped
2		garlic cloves, finely chopped
2	oz.	oil
1–2	cups	veggies (fresh or frozen peas, green beans, carrots, cauliflower)
1	tsp.	salt
1	stick	cinnamon
¾	tsp.	cumin seeds
4		cardamom pods (lightly crushed)
¼	tsp.	turmeric powder
½	tsp.	garam masala
¼	cup	raisins (sultana or regular)
		few slivers of peeled fresh ginger root (or can substitute few dashes ginger powder)
¼	cup	roasted cashews (optional)
1	pinch	ground cloves (optional)

1. Place rice in a strainer and rinse with cold water until water runs clear.

2. Place rice in a bowl and cover with cold water. Let soak for 20 minutes.

3. Drain rice and set aside.

4. In a large saucepan, place oil and add onions and garlic. Sauté 4–5 minutes or until soft.

5. Add ginger, cinnamon, cumin, cardamom, cloves and stir for 2 minutes.

6. Add in the veggies and sauté for 5 minutes.

7. Add the drained rice, salt, turmeric, and garam, raisins, and sauté for 5 minutes.

8. Then, add the water, bring to a boil, and simmer covered for 15–20 minutes (don't overcook rice).

9. Remove from heat and add cashews. Let sit for 5 minutes, then serve.

Mung Dal
Serves 4–6

2½ cups total of:	
	cauliflower, green beans, yellow squash, carrots, and potatoes, and a few leaves of spinach greens
1¾ cups	mung dal
3¾ cups	water (more if needed)
2¾ Tbs.	oil
¾ tsp.	cumin seeds
¾ tsp.	black mustard seeds
¼ tsp.	turmeric
½ tsp.	salt
¾ tsp.	garam masala
½ cup	chopped cilantro
5½ tsp.	minced ginger

1. Wash and chop the vegetables into bite size pieces.

2. Rinse the dal in a strainer 3 or 4 times.

3. Put the rinsed dal and water in a large pot. Bring to a boil and

turn down to a simmer for 15 minutes, stirring frequently.

4. After 15 minutes, add the potatoes, carrots and cauliflower.

5. After another 5 minutes add the squash and green beans. Stir frequently.

6. Continue to cook until the dal and the vegetables are tender, about another 15–20 minutes.

7. Add the greens.

8. Heat the oil in a skillet. Add the mustard and cumin seeds. Stir until the seeds pop.

9. Mix in the cilantro and ginger. Cook for a few minutes, then add the turmeric, salt, and garam masala.

10. Add the oil and spices to the dal and vegetables.

6. Vegetable Stroganoff

Serves 6

3	boxes soft silken tofu
4 Tbs.	balsamic vinegar
1 tsp.	sea salt
1 tsp.	tamari
1 cup	chopped onion
½ lb.	finely chopped mushrooms
2 Tbs.	olive oil
6	cups chopped, steamed vegetable—may include broccoli, cauliflower, carrots, zucchini, peppers, celery, cabbage, and cherry tomatoes
4 cups	whole wheat noodles, cooked and drained (or Explore Asian's Edamame & Mung Bean Fettucine noodles) black pepper to taste

1. Mix tofu, vinegar, salt, tamari, and black pepper in a bowl with a hand blender until smooth and creamy.

2. Sauté onion and mushrooms with olive oil in saucepan until onion is soft.

3. Add tofu mixture and heat through over low flame, stirring regularly. Set aside. May be made ahead of time and reheated before serving.

4. Mix half the sauce with noodles and arrange noodles on a platter with steamed vegetable on top. Serve hot.

Additional sauce maybe served on the side or over the vegetables and noodles

7. Hearty Minestrone Soup & Whole Grain Bread

Serves 4–5

1	cup	white beans (Great Northern or navy)
1½	Tbs.	olive oil
2–3	cups	vegetable broth or bouillon (or you can use just water)
2	cups	tomatoes, whole, diced
½	cup	zucchini, diced
½	cup	yellow squash, diced
½	cup	green beans, cut into 1" pieces
½	cup	carrots, peeled and diced
½	cup	potatoes, scrubbed and diced
1		medium onion, diced
1		clove garlic, minced
½	tsp.	basil dried (or 1 Tbs. fresh)
½	tsp.	oregano
½	tsp.	parsley dried (or 1 Tbs. fresh)
¼	cup	whole grain or soy elbow macaroni
		salt and pepper to taste

1. Cook the macaroni ahead of time, drain, and set aside.

2. If you use dried white beans, soak them in water for 8 hours (or overnight) prior to preparing the soup. Otherwise, you can use canned beans.

3. To cook, first rinse beans and then cook them in fresh water until almost soft, which can take an hour or longer (depending on how fresh the beans are).

4. Heat oil in a large pot over medium-low heat. Add garlic in hot oil and sauté a few minutes.

5. Add onion and cook until slightly softened, 3 to 4 minutes.

6. Stir in carrots and potatoes and sauté for a few minutes.

7. Add broth and diced tomatoes into the onion mixture and bring to a boil, stirring frequently.

8. Reduce the heat to low, and stir in the white beans, green beans, zucchini, squash, tomato, basil, oregano, parsley, salt, and black pepper. Bring to a simmer and then reduce heat so vegetables simmer until tender, about 30 minutes. You can add water as necessary, but the soup should be thick.

9. Just before serving, add in the cooked pasta and stir well. You can always adjust the recipe to your taste, adding more or less veggies.

Can also be served with rice cakes, crackers, or bread.

DESSERT RECIPES

1. Rice Crispy Cashew Treats

Yields approximately 8 squares

4 cups	crispy brown rice cereal (try Erewhon brand as it's sweetened with brown rice syrup vs. sugar)
½ cup	cashew butter
½ cup	maple syrup
⅓ cup	unsweetened shredded coconut (medium shred works best)
2 tsp.	vanilla

1. Add the cashew butter, maple syrup, and vanilla to a saucepan and place on a medium heat.

2. Using a whisk, stir the mixture continuously until it's smooth and hot.

3. Add the coconut and mix well.

4. Remove the mixture from stove and add in the crispy rice, stirring until all the cereal is coated with the mixture.

5. Once coated, you can transfer it to an 8-inch square baking pan (use non-stick pan or place parchment paper in a stainless steel baking pan).

6. Press the mixture down (using the back of a spoon or clean hands) so that it is well packed down and even.

7. Let this cool completely and then cut into the desired number of squares.

2. Miniature Peanut Butter and Jelly Cookies

Yields about 3 dozen

1 cup	whole wheat flour
½ tsp.	baking soda
¾ cup	smooth peanut butter (many health food markets have freshly ground peanut butter or you can grind your own and thus avoid added salt and sugar)
½ cup	maple syrup
1 tsp.	non-alcohol vanilla
⅛ tsp.	sea salt (optional, but may be needed if you are using unsalted peanut butter)
2 Tbs.	strawberry or red raspberry jam

1. Preheat the oven to 350°F.

2. Line two cookie sheets with parchment paper (aluminum foil-backed parchment is ideal as it helps the paper to stick to the baking sheets—parchment side up).

3. Combine the flour, baking soda, and sea salt in a medium size mixing bowl.

4. In a smaller bowl combine the peanut butter, maple syrup, and vanilla. Whisk well, then add to the medium bowl, mixing until well combined.

5. Roll the dough into tiny balls, place on a baking sheet and press your pinky in the center of each cookie.

6. Fill each indentation with a ¼ teaspoon of the jam.

7. Bake for 6–8 minutes or until very lightly browned. Let the cookies cool completely before you remove them from the pan.

3. Tofu Almond Cream with Fresh Fruit

Serves 8–10

1 cup	soft silken tofu
½ cup	maple syrup
½ cup	almond butter
1 tsp.	vanilla extract
1 pinch	sea salt
	fresh juice as needed

1. Combine all of the ingredients in blender until creamy.

2. Add juice for a thinner consistency.

Serve with fresh fruit, cookies, or as a topping on pie.

4. Ginger Carrot Cake

Yields one, 8-inch square or 9-inch round cake

¾	cup	unfiltered apple juice
½	cup	safflower oil
1½	cups	raisins
½	cup	maple syrup
1½	cups	grated carrots (about 3 carrots)
2	tsp.	finely grated ginger
2	cups	whole wheat pastry flour
1	tsp.	baking powder
1	tsp.	baking soda
1	tsp.	cinnamon
½	tsp.	grated nutmeg
½	tsp.	sea salt
1	cup	coarsely chopped walnuts
		zest of 1 orange

1. Preheat oven to 350°.

2. Lightly oil a cake pan, dusting with flour, and removing excess.

3. Mix apple juice, oil, ½ of the raisins, maple syrup, and zest; blend until smooth.

4. Add carrots and ginger and pulse to blend gently.

5. In a large bowl, mix all dry ingredients.

6. Add apple juice mixture and combine with as few strokes as possible. Add remaining raisins and walnuts.

7. Pour into pan, spread evenly with a spatula, and bake until a toothpick inserted into the middle comes out clean, about 40–45 minutes.

5. Rice Pudding

Serves 4

1 cup	short-grain brown rice
1	fresh vanilla bean
1 Tbs.	grated orange zest
¼ tsp.	salt
3 cups	coconut milk
⅓ cup	agave nectar

1. In a small saucepan simmer the rice in 2½ cups water with vanilla bean and orange zest, until liquid is absorbed—15 to 20 minutes.

2. Add milk and sweetener, stirring. Bring up to an easy boil then reduce heat and simmer, stirring frequently, until thick but still a little soupy, about 30 minutes.

3. Taste for sweetness, adding more sweetener if needed.

6. Outrageous Oatmeal Cookies

Yields 3 dozen

1	cup	Earth Balance (non-dairy butter substitute)
1	cup	agave nectar
¼	cup	maple syrup
2		egg replacers
1	tsp.	vanilla
1½	cups	whole wheat pastry flour or soy flour
1	tsp.	baking soda
1	tsp.	cinnamon
¼	tsp.	allspice
¼	tsp.	ground ginger
⅛	tsp.	ground cloves
⅛	tsp.	nutmeg
½	tsp.	salt
3	cups	oats
1	cup	raisins
1	cup	chopped pecans (optional)

1. Heat oven to 350 degrees.
2. Beat together Earth Balance and agave until creamy.
3. Add egg replacer and vanilla. Beat well.
4. Add flour, baking soda, spices, and salt. Mix well.
5. Stir in oats, raisins and nuts. Mix well.
6. Drop by rounded teaspoons on ungreased cookie sheet.
7. Bake 10–12 minutes.

7. Divine Date-Nut Treats

1½   cups total of:
            walnuts, pecans, cashews, or almonds
            (or a combination)
¼   cup   raw sunflower seeds
¾   cup   pitted dates (medjool) soaked overnight, in 1
            cup of water (drain liquid and reserve if needed
            later to make a smoother mixture)
½   cup   maple syrup
¼   cup   cacao or carob powder
½   cup   almond or cashew butter (or a combination)
½   tsp.   non-alcohol vanilla extract

Use to coat:

1–2   cups   finely shredded coconut (unsweetened)
¼   cup   hemp seeds

1. Pulse the walnuts, or nut combination into a food processor until coarsely ground.

2. Add the dates and pulse until well combined with the nuts.

3. Add the rest of the ingredients until the mixture is thick and almost smooth, adding a little soaking water, if needed.

4. Form into golf ball size balls with slightly wet hands

5. Roll half of the batch in coconut and the other half into hemp seeds.

6. Place in a sealed container in the refrigerator to harden or freeze.

These treats are nutritiously good as a snack or a dessert.

QUICK FIX, KID-FRIENDLY MINI-MEAL AND SNACK RECIPES

Note: These are convenience foods chosen for ease of preparation and that require mindful choices on the part of adults not to be given too often to kids, our most precious family members.

1. *Veggie Burgers on Whole Wheat Bun + Sweet Potato Fries*

The new "Bull" burgers are good as are the Gardein brand. Alexia makes a good product for using frozen potatoes and their sweet potato fries, including Cajun style, is excellent. Other suggested brands of burgers are Amy's, and 365 brand (Whole Foods Market's brand). The Gardein brand of beefless sliders are a great fast meal for kids and grown ups alike!

2. *Mock Turkey Sandwiches on Whole Grain Bread*

Suggested brand is Tofurky/Oven Roasted Savory flavor. Another choice of plant based mock meats is the Yves brand. Caution: Many of these type of products contain high salt content which can be excessive in our children's diets. Check those numbers, compared to the protein yield, to make an informed decision.

3. Tofu Dogs on Whole Grain Buns + Rosemary Potatoes

Lightlife makes a fine veg hotdog product as well as Yves, which comes in jumbo and regular sizes. Alexia brand is good, if using frozen potatoes. Naturally processed sauerkraut packs a good probiotic dose, which aids the digestive system. Carefully chosen natural mustard adds flavor without chemical additives.

4. Mock Tuna Salad on Whole Grain Bread

Make your own veg tuna salad or purchase store-bought—but check ingredients since many supermarket brands have egg whites added. These may be labeled as mock "chicken" or "turkey." Some that are made from tempeh have abundant protein. A nice alternative to bread is to use whole grain pita stuffed with the mock tuna. Offer cherry tomatoes & carrot sticks as a side.

Homemade Mock Tuna:

3 cups	Texturized Soy Protein (TSP) or Textured Vegetable Protein (TVP)
3 cups	warm water
1 stalk	celery, minced
½ cup	chopped green pepper
¾ cup	Vegenaise (vegan mayo-type spread)

1. Soak TSP in the warm water for 20–30 minutes.
2. After soaking, squeeze out all excess water.
3. Add the minced celery and Vegenaise and mix well.
4. Optional: add ¼ cup grated onion or "down South" option of ½ cup of pickle relish.

5. Gardein Crispy "Chicken" Tenders

These Gardein brand tenders have the texture and flavor that kids love. Look for good condiments without too much sugar or salt. Beyond Meat brand has three different flavors of mock chicken strips, which are pre-cooked and ready to heat and serve. Convenience at your fingertips!

6. Seasoned Organic Popcorn

Note: This is a truly wonderful whole grain snack, especially when air-popped, which is the healthiest way to prepare popcorn. Try homemade with salt-free popcorn seasonings. Adding nutritional yeast can boost the nutrition. The inexpensive hot air popping machines eliminate the need for oil, making it a healthier snack for the kids. Red Mill makes a good brand of ready-to-pop kernels. Whole Foods' 365 brand makes individual small packets of already popped popcorn that has less fat and sodium than other brands and is organic. These are handy for lunch boxes. Also recommended are two other brands: Skinny and Half Naked popcorn.

7. Frozen Desserts & Fruits

The varieties available today are endless. So Delicious brand soymilk or coconut milk frozen desserts have less sugar than other brands. They also make dairy-free ice cream sandwiches and almond-coated pops. The Tofutti brand of "Cuties" are good child-size portions and delicious. Almond Dream makes mini-sized chocolate-covered "Bites" that are satisfying. Also look for the non-sugar varieties of frozen fruit type sorbets with or without the stick. You can purchase a kit of plastic tray and pop holders and make up your own frozen fruit concoctions sugar-free and delectably refreshing to delight the youngsters.

Happy Healthy Eating!

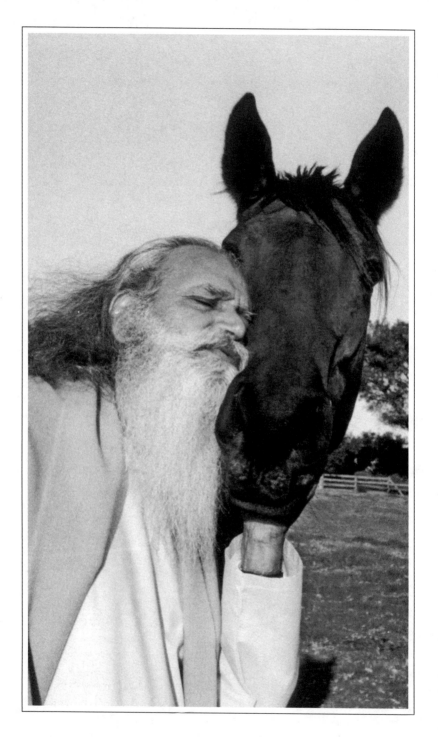

About the Author

Sri Swami Satchidananda was one of the great Yoga masters to bring the classical Yoga tradition to the Western world in the 1960s. He taught Yoga postures and meditation, and he introduced students to a vegetarian diet and a more compassionate lifestyle.

During this period of cultural awakening, iconic pop artist Peter Max, and a small circle of his artist friends, invited Swami Satchidananda to extend an intended two-day visit to New York City so that they could learn from him the secret of experiencing physical health, mental peace, and spiritual enlightenment.

Three years later, he led some half a million American youth in chanting "Om," when he delivered the official opening remarks at the 1969 Woodstock Music and Art Festival and became known as "the Woodstock Guru."

The distinctive teachings that he brought with him blend the physical discipline of Yoga, the spiritual philosophy of India, and the interfaith ideals he pioneered. These techniques and concepts influenced a generation and spawned a Yoga culture that is flourishing today. Currently, over twenty million Americans practice Yoga as a means for managing stress, promoting health, slowing down the aging process, and creating a more meaningful life.

The teachings of Swami Satchidananda have spread into the mainstream, with over 30 Integral Yoga Institutes and Centers on six continents. The Integral Yoga global community includes over 5,000 Integral Yoga teachers—many of whom have become leaders in the changing paradigm of modern Yoga and healthcare, as well as founding successful programs for specific populations. Integral Yoga-inspired programs include Dr. Dean Ornish's landmark work in reversing heart disease, Dr. Michael Lerner's noted Commonweal Cancer Help program, Sonia Sumar's Yoga for the Special Child™, and Rev. Jivana Heyman's Accessible Yoga, among many others.

In 1979, Swami Satchidananda was inspired to establish Satchidananda Ashram–Yogaville in central Virginia. Founded on his teachings, it is a place where people of different faiths and backgrounds can come to realize their essential oneness.

One of the focal points of Yogaville is the Light Of Truth Universal Shrine (LOTUS). This unique interfaith shrine honors the Spirit that unites all the world's faiths, while it celebrates their diversities. People from all over the world come there to meditate and pray. On the occasion of his birth centennial in 2014, a second LOTUS was opened at Swami Satchidananda's birthplace in South India.

Swami Satchidananda served on the advisory boards of many Yoga, world peace, and interfaith organizations. Over the years, he received many honors for his humanitarian service, including the Juliet Hollister Award presented at the United Nations and in 2002, the U Thant Peace Award. In 2014, he was posthumously honored as an "interfaith visionary," with the James Parks Morton Interfaith Award by the Interfaith Center of New York.

Swami Satchidananda is the author of numerous books, while his translation and commentary on *The Yoga Sutras of Patanjali*, the foundation of Yoga philosophy, is the best-selling book of its kind. He is also the subject of the documentary, *Living Yoga: The Life and Teachings of Swami Satchidananda*.

For more information, visit: www.integralyoga.org

About the Contributors

Sandra Amrita McLanahan, M.D.

Dr. McLanahan is a nationally recognized authority on preventive medicine, nutrition, stress reduction, and primary family health care. She founded the nation's first integrative health clinic in 1975 in Connecticut, which was later featured in *Prevention* magazine. As Director of Stress Management Training at the Preventive Medicine Research Institute for twenty years, she worked with Dr. Dean Ornish to document the benefits of dietary change and stress management to prevent and treat cardiovascular disease and cancer. Dr. McLanahan is the author of the book *Surgery and its Alternatives: How to Make the Right Choices for Your Health* and is the medical consultant for the book, *Dr. Yoga*.

Carole Kalyani Baral, M.S.

Carole Kalyani Baral has been a student of Swami Satchidananda since 1973. She received her first Yoga Teaching Certification at the Integral Yoga Institue of New York in 1976 and the second in the "Yoga of the Heart" Training with Nischala Devi in 2010. Carole teaches an Accessible Yoga class in Santa Barbara, California. She has been an avid vegetarian for 40 years and a passionate vegan since 2010. Influenced greatly by the North American Vegetarian Society, she taught Yoga classes and culinary topics for over 35 years at their Summerfest Vegan Conferences. She serves as a member of the Society's Board of Directors.

Reverend Sandra Kumari de Sachy, Ed.D.

Rev. Kumari de Sachy has been practicing Integral Yoga since 1980. She became a certified Integral Yoga teacher in 1981 and was ordained as an Integral Yoga minister in 1995. She has taught Hatha Yoga, Yoga philosophy, and meditation in colleges and universities, in Yoga centers and in prisons, and she continues to teach and serve at Satchidananda Ashram–Yogaville. Kumari has taught English in colleges and universities in the US and in France. She is the author of *Bound to be Free: The Liberating Power of Prison Yoga*, *A Vision of Peace: The Interfaith Teachings of Sri Swami Satchidananda*, and has published a number of articles on Yoga philosophy.

Reverend Prem Anjali, PhD.

Rev. Prem Anjali is an Integral Yoga minister and served as Swami Satchidananda's personal and traveling assistant for 24 years. She is the editorial director for Integral Yoga Publications and *Integral Yoga Magazine*, creative director for Integral Yoga Media, and senior archivist for Integral Yoga Archives. She produced the documentary *Living Yoga: The Life and Teachings of Swami Satchidananda* and is the editor of several books about Swami Satchidananda, including *Portrait of a Modern Sage* and *Boundless Giving*. Prem is the coordinator of the US branch of Service in Satchidananda and was a founding staff member of Integral Health Services, America's first integrative health center.